Women and Mental Disorders

Recent Titles in
Women's Psychology

"Intimate" Violence against Women: When Spouses, Partners, or Lovers Attack
Paula K. Lundberg-Love and Shelly L. Marmion, editors

Daughters of Madness: Growing Up and Older with a Mentally Ill Mother
Susan Nathiel

Psychology of Women: Handbook of Issues and Theories, Second Edition
Florence L. Denmark and Michele Paludi, editors

WomanSoul: The Inner Life of Women's Spirituality
Carole A. Rayburn and Lillian Comas-Diaz, editors

The Psychology of Women at Work: Challenges and Solutions for Our Female Workforce
Michele A. Paludi, editor

Feminism and Women's Rights Worldwide, Three Volumes
Michele A. Paludi, editor

Single Mother in Charge: How to Successfully Pursue Happiness
Sandy Chalkoun

Women and Mental Disorders

Volume 2
Roots in Abuse, Crime, and Sexual Victimization

Paula K. Lundberg-Love, Kevin L. Nadal, and Michele A. Paludi, Editors

Foreword by Ellen Cole

Women's Psychology
Michele A. Paludi, Series Editor

PRAEGER

AN IMPRINT OF ABC-CLIO, LLC
Santa Barbara, California • Denver, Colorado • Oxford, England

Copyright 2012 by Paula K. Lundberg-Love, Kevin L. Nadal, and Michele A. Paludi

All rights reserved. No part of this publication may be reproduced, stored in a retrieval system, or transmitted, in any form or by any means, electronic, mechanical, photocopying, recording, or otherwise, except for the inclusion of brief quotations in a review, without prior permission in writing from the publisher.

Library of Congress Cataloging-in-Publication Data

Women and mental disorders / Paula K. Lundberg-Love, Kevin L. Nadal, and Michele A. Paludi, editors.
 v. ; cm. — (Women's psychology)
Includes bibliographical references and index.
ISBN 978-0-313-39319-8 (hard back : alk. paper) — ISBN 978-0-313-39320-4 (ebook)
1. Women—Psychology. 2. Mental illness. I. Lundberg-Love, Paula K. II. Nadal, Kevin L. III. Paludi, Michele Antoinette.
HQ1206.W8727 2012
362.196'890082—dc23   2011035616

ISBN: 978-0-313-39319-8
EISBN: 978-0-313-39320-4

16 15 14 13 12   1 2 3 4 5

This book is also available on the World Wide Web as an eBook.
Visit www.abc-clio.com for details.

Praeger
An Imprint of ABC-CLIO, LLC

ABC-CLIO, LLC
130 Cremona Drive, P.O. Box 1911
Santa Barbara, California 93116-1911

This book is printed on acid-free paper ∞

Manufactured in the United States of America

I dedicate this book set to all of the women who have struggled to resolve the myriad psychological challenges that we all have encountered during the course of our lives, to the women who not only survived those experiences but thrived in spite of them and thereby created a better human existence. And to all of the women who have given me the opportunity to accompany them on their powerful therapeutic journeys, these volumes are both of you and for you.

Paula K. Lundberg-Love

I dedicate this book set to the fierce and fabulous women who have made my life complete: my mother, my lolas, my aunties, my cousins, my teachers, my mentors, my students, and my dear friends. I also dedicate this book to women everywhere. May their spirits, passion, and love continue to make the world go around.

Kevin L. Nadal

I dedicate this book set to older women who were silenced and labeled as crazy during their lifetimes and to younger women to encourage them to continue to challenge the mental health establishment in honor of their foremothers.

Michele A. Paludi

The criterion of mental health is not one of an individual adjustment to a given social order, but a universal one, valid for all . . . , of giving a satisfactory answer to the problem of human existence.

Erich Fromm

Adult women, all of us, have to come to grips with how we have been affected by gender norms, and how we have been silenced. We have to help our daughters. Understanding it within ourselves and helping our young girls stand up for themselves is one way.

Jane Fonda

Contents

Series Foreword ix
   Michele A. Paludi

Foreword xi
   Ellen Cole

Acknowledgments xiii

Introduction xv
   Michele A. Paludi, Paula K. Lundberg-Love, and
   Kevin L. Nadal

1. Stranger and Acquaintance Rape: Cultural Constructions, Reactions, and Victim Experiences 1
   Beth A. Watson, Kelly A. Kovack, and Maureen C. McHugh

2. Sexual Abuse of Girls and the Lasting Effects 23
   Wesley S. Parks, Paula K. Lundberg-Love, and
   Desiree L. Glaze

3. Women Diagnosed with HIV/AIDS: Experiences of Abuse, Victimization, and Discrimination 43
   Julie Ramos and Kevin L. Nadal

4. Verbal Sexual Coercion in Young Adult Heterosexual Dating Relationships 53
   Jennifer Katz, Vanessa Tirone, and Melanie Schukrafft

5. Intimate Partner Violence as Workplace Violence: Impact on Women's Mental Health and Work Performance 71
   Michele A. Paludi

6. The Effects of Sexism, Gender Microaggressions, and Other Forms of Discrimination on Women's Mental Health and Development 87
   Kevin L. Nadal and Kristal Haynes

7. Sexual Orientation Hate Crimes and the Experiences of LGBT Women 103
   Katie E. Griffin and David A. Schuberth

8. Abuse in Adulthood 121
   William E. Schweinle

9. Intimate Partner Violence during Adolescence 135
   Emilio Ulloa, Vanessa Watts, Monica Ulibarri, Donna Castañeda, and Audrey Hokoda

10. A Feminist Identity Development Model for Filipina Americans: The Influences of Discrimination on Psychological Well-Being and Self-Esteem 163
    Kevin L. Nadal

Appendix: Organizations Dealing with Sexual Victimization and Discrimination of Women 173
Michele A. Paludi

Index 177

About the Editors and Contributors 187

Series Foreword

Michele A. Paludi

Because women's work is never done and is underpaid or unpaid or boring or repetitious and we're the first to get fired and what we look like is more important than what we do and if we get raped it's our fault and if we get beaten we must have provoked it and if we raise our voices we're nagging bitches and if we enjoy sex we're nymphos and if we don't we're frigid and if we love women it's because we can't get a "real" man and if we ask our doctor too many questions we're neurotic and/or pushy and if we expect childcare we're selfish and if we stand up for our rights we're aggressive and "unfeminine" and if we don't we're typical weak females and if we want to get married we're out to trap a man and if we don't we're unnatural and because we still can't get an adequate safe contraceptive but men can walk on the moon and if we can't cope or don't want a pregnancy we're made to feel guilty about abortion and . . . for lots of other reasons we are part of the women's liberation movement.

Author unknown, quoted in The Torch,
September 14, 1987

This sentiment underlies the major goals of Praeger's book series Women's Psychology:

1. *Valuing women.* The books in this series value women by valuing children and working for affordable child care; valuing women by respecting all physiques, not just placing value on slender women; valuing women by acknowledging older women's wisdom, beauty, and aging; valuing women

who have been sexually victimized and viewing them as survivors; valuing women who work inside and outside of the home; and valuing women by respecting their choices of careers, whom they mentor, reproductive rights, spirituality, and sexuality.
2. *Treating women as the norm.* The books in this series make up for women's issues typically being omitted, trivialized, or dismissed from other books on psychology.
3. *Taking a non-Eurocentric view of women's experiences.* The books in this series integrate the scholarship on race and ethnicity into women's psychology, thus providing a psychology of *all* women. Women typically have been described collectively, but we are diverse.
4. *Facilitating connections between readers' experiences and psychological theories and empirical research.* The books in this series offer readers opportunities to challenge their views about women, feminism, sexual victimization, gender role socialization, education, and equal rights. These texts thus encourage women readers to value themselves and others. The accounts of women's experiences as reflected through research and personal stories in the texts in this series have been included for readers to derive strength from the efforts of others who have worked for social change on the interpersonal, organizational, and societal levels.

A student in one of my courses on the psychology of women once stated:

> I learned so much about women. Women face many issues: discrimination, sexism, prejudices . . . by society. Women need to work together to change how society views us. I learned so much and talked about much of the issues brought up in class to my friends and family. My attitudes have changed toward a lot of things. I got to look at myself, my life, and what I see for the future. (Paludi, 2002)

It is my hope that readers of the books in this series will also reflect on the topics and look at themselves, their own lives, and what they see for the future.

The four-volume set *Women and Mental Disorders* provides readers with the opportunity to accomplish this goal and offers suggestions for psychotherapists, career counselors, academicians, attorneys, and health professionals who work with women. This set also assists us as advocates in guiding institutional and social policy change in work and educational institutions and in lobbying state and federal legislators on issues related to women and mental health, especially violence against women.

REFERENCE

Paludi, M. (2002). *The psychology of women* (2nd ed.). Upper Saddle River, NJ: Prentice Hall.

Foreword

Ellen Cole

Many of the readers of this four-volume book set will be too young to recall that it was Carol Hanisch, a radical feminist from New York City, who popularized the phrase "the personal is political" in a 1969 essay with the same title. I am reminded of that phrase today and its offshoot, "the political is personal," as I sit here to write this foreword on March 9, 2011, sandwiched between a day that is political yet personal and a day that is personal yet political. You see, yesterday we celebrated the 100th anniversary of International Women's Day. Tomorrow, March 10, I turn 70.

The first International Women's Day was held in 1911 in Germany, Austria, Denmark, and Switzerland. Today it is a worldwide annual event that continues to honor women's achievements, educate about the importance and worth of women in society, and raise awareness of both gains made and injustices, atrocities, and violence against women still to be overcome.

Clearly, many gains have been made since 1911. Economic opportunities, political participation, and educational attainment for women are vastly improved. And yet recent headlines scream at us that our work is far from done. A recent White House report, for example, states that men still get paid more to do the same jobs as women (in 2009 women made on average 75% of what their male counterparts earned), and women are more likely than men to live in poverty. Sex trafficking is called the new slavery. We read reports about women in Afghanistan who are set on fire or who set themselves on fire to escape impossible lives or about women being held in U.S. custody, awaiting trial or deportation, who are sexually assaulted by male guards. The list is long. The political is personal.

Tomorrow I turn 70. I have lived through the second wave of feminism and its many offspring. I've seen the development of women's studies and gender studies as respected academic disciplines and the development of feminist psychology and feminist therapy. I've seen the movement embrace and then be led by women of color and lesbian, bisexual, and transgender women. I've seen new foci emerge and become front and center in feminist scholarship: multiculturalism and diversity, social justice and social action, and feminist collaboration, process, and leadership, to name a few. I feel incredibly fortunate to have been able to participate in what may be the revolution of the century, that of the rights of women and girls. But it is a revolution that is far from complete. The personal is political.

I want to commend the editors and the authors of this four-volume book set. They tackle it all (I say this with forethought), stating their major goals as valuing women, treating women as the norm, coming from a non-Eurocentric perspective, and connecting theory, research, and women's experience. The author list reads like a who's who in women's mental health and feminist psychology. The topics are current and far-ranging. If you would like to know more about women with disabilities, the feminization of poverty, psychological well-being for women, microaggressions against women, women and spirituality, reproduction, hate crimes, intimate partner abuse, specific disorders (e.g., agoraphobia, eating disorders, borderline personality disorder, sexual dysfunction, teenage cutting), or a variety of approaches to treatment and research, you will find it and much more in the pages of these four volumes. It is exhilarating to know that they are available as resources for all of us in education, health, social policy, and more who work with women. I am grateful to the editors and authors for the timeliness of this contribution. Two days ago, Secretary of State Hillary Rodham Clinton told a *Newsweek* reporter that "I believe that the rights of women and girls is the unfinished business of the 21st century." I agree, and the chapters in this book set help us move toward finishing that business.

Acknowledgments

Editing these volumes with Michele Paludi and Kevin Nadal has been an enriching experience, and I hope it is the first of many. Having the support and dedication of Debbie Caravalko at Praeger as a mentor is always a rewarding endeavor. The wide range of expertise of all of the contributors made this project a stimulating and enriching one. I also want to acknowledge three people who have supported me in this project in spite of obstacles encountered by them, namely my colleague Andrew Schmitt and my accomplished graduate students Wes Parks and Desiree Glaze. Thank you for your commitment and your dedication.

Also noteworthy are the people who serve as my inspiration when I engage in an endeavor such as this. They are my wonderful daughter Jill Wright and my two irrepressible granddaughters, Lexi and Lily Wright. I hope that books such as this one inspire them.

However, the person who has probably supported me the most in my scholarly endeavors and believed in me since our journey through graduate school is my friend Michele Paludi. Thank you Michele for all of the enrichment that you have generously provided to so many women.

Paula K. Lundberg-Love

I thank Michele Paludi and Paula Lundberg-Love for giving me the opportunity to edit this book set. I am looking forward to a future of collaborative efforts. I thank my family and friends, who have always been supportive of my career and my passion for social justice. I especially thank my parents, my brothers, my sister; the Yabut, Nadal, and Tamayo clans; and Randy Fabellore. And finally, I thank all of the contributors for their expertise and fervor. We need more people like you to advocate for the marginalized and to give voice to those who are silenced.

Kevin L. Nadal

I thank Paula Lundberg-Love and Kevin Nadal for the opportunity to collaborate with them on this book set. Our collaboration has been a wonderful experience for me. I also acknowledge the support and caring from the following people during the preparation of this book set: Rosalie Paludi, Lucille Paludi, Carmen Paludi Jr., Cay Raycroft, and David Raycroft. Working with Debbie Carvalko at Praeger again has been rewarding. I thank her for her encouragement, mentoring, and support.

I also have learned a great deal from the contributors to this book set. Thank you for being part of this project. Your work has strengthened our understanding of women and mental disorders.

Michele A. Paludi

Introduction

Michele A. Paludi, Paula K. Lundberg-Love, and Kevin L. Nadal

CLAUDIA: *NUTS?*

> The ethic of mental health is masculine in our culture. This double standard of sexual mental health, which exists side by side with a single and masculine standard of *human* mental health, is enforced by both society and clinicians. Although the limited "ego resources," and unlimited "dependence," and fearfulness of most women is pitied, disliked, and "diagnosed," by society and its agent-clinicians, any other kind of behavior is unacceptable in women!
>
> Phyllis Chesler (*Women and Madness,* 1972, p. 69)

In *Nuts,* Tom Topor's play that was later adapted to the screen (starring Barbra Streisand and directed by Martin Ritt), the protagonist, Claudia Draper, is confined to a mental hospital by her parents in an effort to keep her from standing trial for the murder of a client. The play and movie depict Claudia, a high-class escort, in court fighting for her right to stand trial for manslaughter rather than being declared mentally incompetent. Kempley (1987, p. 3) stated that *Nuts* has the purpose of "pitting inner truths against outward appearances to force us to decide who is and is not nuts."

During the competency hearing, Claudia states that "I am not just a picture in your heads. I am not just a daughter, or a wife, or a hooker, or a patient or a defendant." She is determined that others not label her or control her life according to their terms, to their perceptions of who they think she is. She speaks up against psychiatrists who don't like her and challenge their authority.

Claudia keeps maintaining that she is sane. As Brussat and Brussat (1987, p. 2) stated, *"Nuts* is a gutsy movie . . . with an unlikable heroine who refuses to submit to the purposes, fantasies, or needs of others." The viewer comes to learn that Claudia was sexually molested by her stepfather for years until she was 16 years old. We further learn that she killed her client in self-defense.

DORA/IDA: MENTALLY ILL?

> The great question that has never been answered and which I have not yet been able to answer, despite my thirty years of research into the feminine soul, is "What does a woman want?"
>
> Sigmund Freud

Nuts in many ways is a retelling of a classic case discussed by Sigmund Freud in his 1905 article "Fragment of an Analysis of a Case of Hysteria." This "case of hysteria" is better known in academic and lay circles as the case of "Dora." Dora (not her real name) was an 18-year-old woman who was brought for treatment to Freud by her father, one of Freud's former patients. Dora's parents were concerned about her based on some recent behavior, including a suicide note. Freud also noted that Dora had a "nervous" cough, a history of fainting spells, headaches, and depression that dated back to her childhood. Dora's "most troubling symptom" for Freud was her "complete loss of voice." Freud diagnosed Dora as a "typical case of hysteria." His goal was to explain to her the sexual meanings of her symptoms: repressed content of her early sexuality, masturbatory fantasies, lesbian fantasies, and incestuous desires for her father.

Freud learned that Dora's father was having an extramarital affair with Frau K., the wife of a family friend, Herr K. Herr K. had attempted to rape Dora, the first time when she was 14 years old. Dora explained that she believed "she had been handed over to Herr K." by her father in exchange for Herr K.'s complicity in the affair. Dora also believed that her father "handed her over" to Freud because he feared that she would discuss the affair. Her father hired Freud to "bring her to reason" (Freud, 1905, pp. 188, 183).

Initially Freud believed Dora's account of why her father had brought her to him for treatment: "I came to the conclusion that Dora's story must correspond to the facts in every respect." Freud noted that Dora's father and Herr K. conspired against her: "Each of the two men avoided drawing any conclusions from the other's behavior which would have been awkward for his own plans" (Freud, 1905, p. 35).

We note, however, that Freud published the case, despite the fact it was incomplete, because he believed that it demonstrated the sexual origins of hysteria. In a critique of Freud's analysis, Showalter (1985, p. 160) noted:

> In his case history of Dora, if not in the actual treatment, Freud is determined to have the last word—he even has a postscript—in constructing

his own "intelligible, consistent, and unbroken" account of her hysteria. He asserts his intellectual superiority to this bright but rebellious young woman. He uses his text to demonstrate his power to bring a woman to reason, and to bring reason to the mysteries of woman.

Similar to what we learn by watching *Nuts,* there is an alternative analysis to Dora's behavior. She was brought to Freud by her father to cast her in a sick role. She was sexually abused by a trusted family friend when she was a young adolescent. And her experiences were relabeled by Freud in order to support his theory of female personality development.

Claudia's parents wanted her committed to a mental hospital because she must be nuts to kill a man and not discuss the sexual abuse by her stepfather that she endured for years (her mother stated that she was unaware of the abuse). Claudia's therapists reinterpreted all of her comments and nonverbal behavior in terms of pathology. Like Dora, Claudia was caught in a web of deceit and betrayal. Also similar to Claudia, Dora's name was changed by Freud. Her real name was Ida Bauer. Claudia kept being referred to by the wrong name, a name given to her in the hearing trial. Williams (1983, p. 42) noted that Freud might have said to Ida, "You are right and they are wrong." Freud did not, however, and Ida continued to have symptoms throughout her adult life.

Cixous (1976) interpreted the case of Dora/Ida in terms of the silencing of women who question patriarchal assumptions. According to Cixous, "Silence is the mark of hysteria. The great hysterics have lost speech . . . their tongues are cut off and what talks isn't heard because it's the body that talks and man doesn't hear the body" (p. 49). Showalter (1985, p. 161) also recognized that women's hysteria fits in well with patriarchy: "Hysteria is tolerated because in fact it has no power to effect cultural change; it is much safer for the patriarchal order to encourage and allow discontented women to express their wrongs through psychosomatic illness than to have them agitating for economic and legal rights."

Thus, women who behave according to social expectations were often considered crazy. As Chesler (1972) noted, being too "feminine" or not "feminine" enough were grounds for being considered mentally ill.

WOMEN: UNHEALTHY ADULTS? THE DOUBLE STANDARD FOR MENTAL HEALTH

> As a feminist therapist, I had had ample opportunity to observe the negative synergy of trauma and silence, abuse and secrecy, that would lead women to feel and act crazy, when in fact it was mainly the context in which they were forced to operate that was pathological.
>
> Laura S. Brown

That there exists a double standard for mental health was demonstrated by Broverman, Broverman, Clarkson, Rosenkrantz, and Vogel (1970), who found that mental health practitioners described characteristics of adult men and adults in a similar manner but differed from the characteristics that they assigned to adult women. Adults and adult men were described by personality characteristics as follows: very direct, very logical, can make decisions easily, and never cry. Adult women were described with the following characteristics: less independent, very illogical, very sneaky, less adventurous, more easily influenced, and very excitable in minor crises. This research suggested that a woman could not be simultaneously described as a healthy woman and a healthy adult. According to Broverman et al., "The general standard of health is actually applied only to men, while healthy women are perceived as significantly less healthy by adult standards" (p. 5).

Women's psychological adjustment has been constructed based on male development. Consequently, feminist theorists and therapists have developed new models of mental health that value women and women's roles (Gilbert, 1999; Russo & Tartaro, 2008; Landrine & Russo, 2009). There have been five priority areas outlined to meet this goal of valuing women in mental health research and treatment (e.g., Eichler & Parron, 1987):

1. Diagnosis and treatment of mental disorders in women.
2. Stressors involved in poverty.
3. Stressors involved in multiple roles of partner, parent, elder caregiver, and employee.
4. Older women's mental health issues.
5. Causes and mental health impact of violence against women.

Each of these priority areas will be briefly addressed below. These areas are also addressed in the four volumes of this book set.

Diagnosis and Treatment of Mental Disorders in Women

Women are diagnosed and treated for mental illness at a higher rate than men (Russo & Tartaro, 2008). Women are more likely than men to be diagnosed as being agoraphobic, having anxiety, being depressed, or having an eating disorder (Desjarlais, Eisenberg, Good, & Kleinman, 1996; Sachs-Ericsson & Ciarlo, 2000). Comorbidity is also higher for women. Women are more likely to have three or more psychiatric disorders in their life cycle (Russo & Tartaro, 2008). Furthermore, according to Russo and Tartaro (2008, p. 449), "Evidence for overpathologizing by psychologists has been in higher probability of overdiagnosis of depression (particularly by male psychiatrists) in women." In addition to overpathologizing mental disorders in women, some disorders such as alcoholism and drug abuse have been underdiagnosed in women (Russo, 1995).

Research has also highlighted the fact that women (especially older women) are more likely than men to be prescribed psychotropic drugs at higher rates

(Hamilton, Grant, & Jensvold, 1996). Yonkers and Hamilton (1995) pointed out that therapists misdiagnose women as being depressed when they may have other disorders that are being relabeled as depression.

Several studies have interpreted the diagnostic labeling as resulting from one of two explanations: (1) women are more likely to exhibit behaviors that men will label as mental illness because women have been socialized to express their emotions or (2) women have unequal social position and experience more discrimination, harassment, and other forms of violence and victimization (Gilbert, 1999; Paludi & Denmark, 2011).

Furthermore, women from different cultures and with varying sexual orientations and gender identities are often misdiagnosed because their social identities do not match that of the majority culture. Thus, it is even more important to recognize how intersectional identities may result in misdiagnoses.

Stressors Involved in Poverty

Women's depressive symptomatology has been explained in part by low-income and ethnic minority or racial minority status (Belle, 1984). Belle, Longfellow, Makosky, Saunders, and Zelkowitz (1981) reported that their sample of 42 urban low-income mothers had personally experienced 37 violent events and witnessed 35 stressful events to friends and family during the previous two years. In addition, Brown (1995) noted that living in dangerous neighborhoods, having financial concerns, and living in inadequate housing are more significant stressors for women than are acute crises. Herd (2009) found that older women are more likely to be living in poverty, noting marriage and public pension benefits as contributing factors to the poverty.

The phrase "feminization of poverty" (Pearce, 1978) refers to more women heads of households who are living below the poverty line. Their experiences result from nonpayment of child support following a divorce and inadequate and/or expensive child care (Gadalla, 2008). Belle (1984) also found that poverty undermines the sources of social support for women that otherwise buffer the impact of stress. Because women are also experiencing stress in their support system, their lives have more stress, and they are therefore at greater risk for depression. White (2010) reported that poverty for women makes them vulnerable to HIV transmission.

Polakoff and Gregory (2002), Fukuda-Parr (1999), and Thibos, Lavin-Loucks, and Martin (2007) noted that the feminization of poverty includes much more than financial need. According to Thibos et al., "being poor also implies the absence of choice, the denial of opportunity, the inability to achieve life goals, and ultimately the loss of hope. Thus, the phenomenon of a feminized poverty extends beyond the economic domains of income and material needs to the core of individual and family life. . . . Indeed, some of the most striking evidence for the prevalence of a feminized poverty is the rate of poverty among children, who disproportionately reside in female-headed households" (p. 1).

Stressors Involved in Multiple Roles of Women

There is an incompatibility between work and family roles. For example:

1. Employed women are more likely to lack fringe benefits needed to care for their family (Paludi & Neidermeyer, 2008).
2. Employed women are more likely to lack job flexibility in order to care for themselves, children, and elderly parents (Paludi et al., 2008).
3. Women face the opportunity gap, factors that bar women from advancing in their careers at the same rate as men (Jandeska & Kraimer, 2005).
4. Salary inequities remain, especially for women of color (Hewlett, 2002).
5. Employed women do substantially more caregiving to children and elderly parents than do men (Heymann, 2000; Strassel, Colgan, & Goodman, 2006).

The incompatibility between the workplace and family demands is exacerbated by a relative lack of provisions that would ease women's integration of these roles. Furthermore, the reality that most children are being raised in single-parent homes has been ignored. In addition, equality of the parenting and housekeeping roles has not been achieved (Flouri & Buchanan, 2002; Strassel et al., 2006). For example, women perform more housework than men, and this applies even for women in academia and the sciences (Hersch, 2009; Milkie, Raley, & Bianchi, 2009). According to research conducted by the United States Department of Labor, Bureau of Labor Statistics (2010):

1. Eighty-four percent of women and 63% of men perform housework.
2. Employed women do approximately twice the amount of child care as employed men (44 minutes versus 23 minutes during a 24-hour period).
3. Dual-career families follow traditional husband-wife roles. Women spend approximately 80 minutes more during a day on home and child care responsibilities while spending 1 hour less at work.

Heymann's (2000) research suggested that there is an impact on children's health when at least one parent is not achieving work/life integration, including:

1. Sick children have shorter recovery periods. They have better vital signs and fewer symptoms when their parents participate in their care.
2. The presence of a parent reduces hospital stays by 31%.
3. Children recover more quickly from outpatient assistance when at least one parent is involved in their care.
4. There is a significant impact on children's educational outcomes when parents are not achieving work/life integration. When parents are involved in their children's education, children achieve more at all grade levels.
5. Children's higher achievement in math and language is associated with the involvement of at least one parent.

6. Teens are less likely to drop out of school if at least one parent is involved in their studying.

Research has identified noted costs to women who integrate work and family roles. For example, employed women who report work/life conflict are as much as 30 times more likely to experience a significant mental health problem, including depression and anxiety, than women who report no such conflict (Gonzalez-Morales, Peiro, & Greenglass, 2006). Psychological symptoms associated with integrating these roles include isolation, guilt, self-consciousness, frustration, alienation, withdrawal from social situations, and decreased self-esteem (Karsten, 2006). Research has also identified a variety of physical health complaints among women integrating multiple roles, including but not limited to headaches, tiredness, lethargy, gastrointestinal disorders, eating disorders, and inability to concentrate.

Research has indicated that maternal employment has been related to positive impacts on children (Han, Waldfogel, & Brooks-Gunn, 2001). For example, daughters of employed mothers are more career oriented (versus home oriented) than daughters of full-time homemakers. In addition, daughters of employed mothers are more likely to pursue nontraditional careers than daughters of full-time homemakers. Maternal employment influences women's career development through its provision of a role model of women's employment (Gottfried, Gottfried, & Bathurst, 2002). Whether the mother is employed is not the most critical factor; rather, it is the mother's role satisfaction and assistance with integrating work/life roles that has the greatest impact on children.

Research has also noted that married women have higher rates of admission to mental health facilities than married men (Russo & Green, 1993). Marecek (1978) suggested that married women may experience a loss of independence and status as well as difficulties associated with the multiple roles of wife, mother, and employee, all of which can create stress and lead to mental illness. Furthermore, women are likely to have a major part of their identity tied to their ability to successfully establish intimate relationships. When the romantic relationship ends, they may experience emotional problems as a result of regarding themselves as a failure in terms of the cultural standards of femininity (Carnelley, Wortman, & Kessler, 1999).

Older Women and Mental Health Issues

Paludi and DeFour (2010) identified the fact that older women are at risk of control by others, including family members, caregivers, and health care workers. Older women experience dependency and a loss of self-reliance due to physical and/or mental impairments. These impairments lead to older women's need for help with even the most basis activities of daily living, including personal hygiene care, maintenance of the home, and handling finances. Furthermore, older women have chronic illnesses and debilitating disorders, including Alzheimer's disease, strokes, and heart disorders, that require care (Etaugh, 2008).

In addition, older women are unable to defend themselves against the impact of abuse and/or neglect. Older women are at increased risk for intimate partner abuse; sexual assault, including marital rape; caregiver abuse; and impaired access to employment or education (Paludi & DeFour, 2010). The impact of this abuse includes permanent physical damage, loss of confidence, confusion, and depression.

In addition, there is a double standard of aging in North American culture (Paludi, 2010; Sontag, 1979). Aging in women alters the qualities of femininity in a culture (e.g., attractiveness, desirability, and reproductive capacity). Since masculinity is identified with independence, autonomy, competency, and self-control, aging does not threaten these qualities (Etaugh, 2008). Consequently, middle-aged and older women are more dissatisfied with age-related physical changes than are middle-aged and older men. Often older women strive to achieve the facial features and physique of younger women through age-concealment techniques in order to be accepted by a culture that values young women (Chrisler, Gorman, Chapman, & Serra, 2010; Digman & Otte, 2010; Frederick, Peplau, & Lever, 2008).

Heilbrun (1991, p. 56) noted that "signs of age come upon women in our society like marks of the devil in earlier times." Older women are informed of the social norms for "appropriate" fashion for their aging female body, including refraining from wearing bright colors; wearing revealing, suggestive styles; and masking body "transgressions" (Pruis & Janowsky, 2010).

CAUSES AND MENTAL HEALTH IMPACT OF VIOLENCE AGAINST WOMEN

Throughout the life cycle, women are victims of violence including rape, intimate partner violence, stalking, child sexual abuse, workplace violence, and sexual harassment (Lundberg-Love & Marmion, 2006). For example, during childhood and adolescence (Paludi & Denmark, 2011):

1. Ten percent of teen girls report they have experienced physical violence in their dating relationships.
2. Seventy-one percent of school-aged girls report being bullied.
3. Between kindergarten and 12th grade, more than 4.5 million children and adolescents are targets of sexual harassment by a teacher, administrator, or other school employee.
4. Approximately 30% of adolescent girls are victims of child sexual abuse.

Paludi (2010) noted that with respect to college women:

1. One in every 20 is raped.
2. Acquaintance rape is more common than stranger rape.

3. Fifty percent to 80% of rape victims know their assailant (Gerber & Cherneski, 2006).
4. Women ages of 16 to 24 are raped at rates four times higher than the assault rate of all women (Fisher, Cullen, & Turner, 2000).
5. Intimate partner violence impacts 10% to 44% of students, including being slapped, having objects thrown at them, or being pushed, grabbed, shoved.

Paludi and DeFour (2010) reported that approximately 1.5 million women between the ages of 45 and 64 are physically abused by their mates, and approximately 1.5 million older women living in institutions are victims of abuse annually.

Research has documented impact on survivors' areas of functioning, including emotional/psychological, physical or health related, career, interpersonal, and self-perception (Dansky & Kilpatrick, 1997; McCann, 2001; Waits & Lundberg-Love, 2008). Examples of emotional/psychological effects of violence include but are not limited to guilt, denial, withdrawal from social settings, depression, fear, anger, isolation, fear of crime in general, helplessness, shock, and decreased self-esteem.

The following are reported physical/health-related effects of violence: headaches, fatigue, respiratory problems, substance abuse, sleep disturbances, eating disorders, lethargy, and gastrointestinal disorders.

Career effects include changes in work habits, absenteeism, and changes in career goals, including leaving school or occupations in order to escape the violence. The impact that violence has on social and interpersonal relationships includes the following: fear of new people, lack of trust, changes in social networks, and withdrawal.

Violence against girls and women has been recognized as a major public health and human rights issue that is explained by unequal power relations and patriarchal values.

FEMINIST THERAPIES

> As a feminist therapist, I am aware that our best work comes out of our experience as women working with women. Only if our theory remains close to and within the world of women can it be a truly woman-based theory. The viewpoint must be female rather than male, as it has usually been.
>
> *Hannah Lerman*

These realities of women's mental health and illness outlined in the five priority areas have implications for psychotherapy for women. Several feminist therapies have been offered to assist women in finding support for issues relating to victimization, aging, poverty, and role conflict (e.g., Gilbert, 1999; Moor, 2010, 2011; Worell, 1980). Feminist therapies accept the idea that society's definitions of gender roles and the devaluation of women and femininity must cease (Marecek & Kravetz, 1998).

The following guidelines endorsed by feminist therapists have been outlined by Worell (1980, pp. 480–481):

1. Providing an egalitarian relationship with shared responsibility between counselor and client. The client is encouraged to trust her own judgment and to arrive at her own decisions. In contrast to many traditional counseling relationships, the client is never in a one-down position of having to accept counselor interpretations of her behavior or external prescriptions for appropriate living.
2. Employing a consciousness-raising approach. Women are helped to become aware of the societal restraints on their development and opportunities. Clients are helped to differentiate between the politics of the sexist social structure and those problems over which they have realistic personal control.
3. Helping women explore a sense of their personal power and how they can use it constructively in personal, business, and political relationships.
4. Helping women to get in touch with unexpressed anger in order to combat depression and to make choices about how to use their anger constructively.
5. Helping women to redefine themselves apart from their role relationships to men, children, and home; exploring women's fears about potential role changes that may alienate spouse and children as well as coworkers and boss.
6. Encouraging women to nurture themselves as well as care for others, thereby raising self-confidence and self-esteem.
7. Encouraging multiple skill development to increase women's competence and productivity. This may include assertiveness training, economic and career skills, and negotiation skills with important others who resist change.

In 2000, the Council of Representatives of the American Psychological Association adopted the Guidelines for Psychotherapy with Lesbian, Gay, and Bisexual Clients. These guidelines including having psychologists "strive to understand the ways in which social stigmatization (e.g., prejudice, discrimination, violence) poses risks to the mental health and well-being of lesbian, gay, and bisexual clients." These guidelines also advise psychologists that homosexuality and bisexuality are not indicative of any mental illness.

Thus, feminist therapists believe that what has been called mental illness needs to be reconsidered (Bravo-Rosewater, 1984; Gilbert, 1999). Bravo-Rosewater recommended that psychotherapists should concentrate not on diagnosis per se but rather on the implications of the diagnosis. According to Bravo-Rosewater:

> If a woman is diagnosed as depressed, what assumptions underlie that label? Is it assumed that women are generally unhappy individuals? Is it assumed that depressed individuals are hopeless? Is the appropriate remedy psychotherapy or chemotherapy or shock treatments? . . . A feminist analysis of depression sees it as originating from women's role in society. . . . A feminist treatment of depression, therefore, centers on an examination of the

environmental impact on the woman in treatment, historically and currently. Depression may be viewed as a coping skill or as a health reaction to an unjust situation. . . . The role expectations for women in our society and whether a given role is right for any particular woman needs to be critically examined. Feminist therapy aids in the reevaluating and renegotiating of specific roles and the rules governing those roles (pp. 272–273).

THE PRESENT BOOK SET

This four-volume set on women and mental disorders features scholarly research about the following major topics: women's unique life experiences (e.g., feminist identity, poverty, spirituality); roots of abuse, crime, and sexual victimization (e.g., date rape, intimate partner violence, hate crimes); common mental disorders (e.g., anorexia, bulimia, agoraphobia); and treatments and research (e.g., counseling girls with eating disorders, ethnocultural psychotherapy, treating depression, histrionic personality disorder, and treatment of substance abuse).

We take a multicultural approach to women and mental disorders, including discussing international migration experiences of Asian women, depression among Caribbean women, international perspectives on women's mental health, and therapeutic needs that vary by women's age, culture, and income. We also offer readers resources on women's mental health and mental disorders.

Thus, this book set addresses the four biases toward women that the field of psychology and psychiatry has held for years (Worell, 1990): androcentrism (the prototype of humankind based on men), gendercentrism (separate paths of development theorized for women and men), ethnocentrism (personality development is identical across national origins and races), and heterosexism (heterosexual orientation is normative). Our goal is that these four volumes stimulate additional research agendas on women and mental disorders and mental health that make all women central, not marginal, as has been done by the early psychoanalytic theorists.

REFERENCES

Belle, D. (1984). Inequality and mental health: Low income and minority women. In L. Walker (Ed.), *Women and mental health policy* (pp. 135–150). Beverly Hills, CA: Sage.

Belle, D., Longfellow, C., Makosky, V., Saunders, E., & Zelkowitz, P. (1981). Income, mothers' mental health and family functioning in a low-income population. In American Academy of Nursing (Ed.), *The impact of changing resources on health policy* (pp. 28–37). Kansas City, MO: American Nurses Association.

Bravo-Rosewater, L. (1984). Feminist therapy: Implications for practitioners. In L. Walker (Ed.), *Women and mental health policy.* Beverly Hills, CA: Sage.

Broverman, I., Broverman, D., Clarkson, F., Rosenkrantz, P., & Vogel, S. (1970). Sex role stereotypes and clinical judgments of mental health. *Journal of Consulting and Clinical Psychology, 34,* 1–7.

Brown, L. (1995). Cultural diversity in feminist therapy: Theory and practice. In H. Landrine (Ed.), *Bringing cultural diversity to feminist psychology* (pp. 143–162). Washington, DC: American Psychological Association.

Brussat, F., & Brussat, M. (1987). *Nuts*. Spirituality and Practice. Retrieved on October 12, 2010, from www.spiritualityandpractice.com/films/films.php?id=9035.

Carnelley, K., Wortman, C., & Kessler, R. (1999). The impact of widowhood on depression: Findings from prospective survey. *Psychological Medicine, 29*, 1111–1123.

Chesler, P. (1972). *Women and madness*. New York: Avon Books.

Chrisler, J., Gorman, J., Chapman, K., & Serra, K. (2010). *Facing up to aging: Women's attitudes toward cosmetic procedures*. Paper presented at the New York Academy of Sciences and Pace University's Conference on Women, Power and Aging, New York City.

Cixous, H. (1976). *Portrait de Dora*. Paris: Editions des femmes.

Dansky, B., & Kilpatrick, D. (1997). Effects of sexual harassment. In W. O'Donohue (Ed.), *Sexual harassment: Theory, research and practice* (pp. 152–174). Boston: Allyn & Bacon.

Desjarlais, R., Eisenberg, L., Good, B., & Kleinman, A. (1996). *World mental health: Problems and priorities in low-income countries*. Oxford: Oxford University Press.

Digman, S., & Otte, M. (2010). *The embodiment of aging in an era of plastic surgery: What does it mean to be old now?* Paper presented at the New York Academy of Sciences and Pace University's Conference on Women, Power and Aging, New York City.

Eichler, A., & Parron, D. (1987). *Women's mental health: Agenda for research*. Rockville, MD: National Institute of Mental Health.

Etaugh, C. (2008). Women in the middle and later years. In F. Denmark & M. Paludi (Eds.), *Psychology of women: A handbook of issues and theories* (pp. 271–302). Westport, CT: Praeger.

Fisher, B., Cullen, F., & Turner, M. (2000). *The sexual victimization of college women*. Washington, DC: U.S. Department of Justice, National Institute of Justice and Bureau of Justice Statistics.

Flouri, E., & Buchanan, A. (2002). What predicts fathers' involvement with their children? A prospective study of intact families. *British Journal of Developmental Psychology, 21*, 81–98.

Frederick, D. A., Peplau, L. A., & Lever, J. (2008). The Barbie mystique: Satisfaction with breast size and shape across the lifespan. *International Journal of Sexual Health, 20*, 200–211.

Freud, Sigmund. (1905). Bruchstück einer Hysterie-Analyse. *Mschr. Psychiat. Neurol., 28*, pp. 285–310, 408–467; *G.W., 5*, pp. 161–286; Fragment of an analysis of a case of hysteria, *SE, 7*, 1–122.

Freud, S. (1963). *Dora: An analysis of a case of hysteria*. Transcribed by James Strachey. New York: Collier.

Fukuda-Parr, S. (1999). What does feminization of poverty mean? It isn't just lack of income. *Feminist Economics, 5*, 99–103.

Gadalla, T. (2008). Gender differences in poverty rates after marital dissolution: A longitudinal study. *Journal of Divorce and Remarriage, 3*, 225–238.

Gerber, G., & Cherneski, L. (2006). Sexual aggression toward women: Reducing the prevalence. In F. Denmark, H. Krauss, E. Halpern, & J. Sechzer (Eds.), *Violence and exploitation against women and girls* (pp. 35–46). Boston: Blackwell.

Gilbert, L. A. (1999). Reproducing gender in counseling and psychotherapy: Understanding the problem and changing the practice. *Applied and Preventative Psychology, 8*, 119–127.

Gonzales-Morales, M., Peiro, J., & Greenglass, E. (2006). Coping and distress in organizations: The role of gender in work stress. *International Journal of Stress Management, 13,* 228–248.

Gottfried, A., Gottfried, A., & Bathurst, K. (2002). Maternal and dual earner employment status and parenting. In M. Bornstein (Ed.), *Handbook of parenting: Vol. 2. Biology and ecology of parenting* (pp. 207–229). Hillsdale, NJ: Erlbaum.

Hamilton, J., Grant, M., & Jensvold, M. (1996). Sex and treatment of depressions: When does it matter? In J. Hamilton, M. Jensvold, E. Rothblum, & E. Cole (Eds.), *Psychopharmacology of women: Sex, gender and hormonal considerations* (pp. 241–260). Washington, DC: American Psychiatric Press.

Han, W., Waldfogel, J. & Brooks-Gunn, J. (2001). The effects of early maternal employment on later cognitive and behavioral outcomes. *Journal of Marriage and the Family, 63,* 336–354.

Heilbrun, C. (1991). *The last gift of time: Life beyond sixty.* New York: Dell.

Herd, P. (2009). Women, public pensions, and poverty: What can the United States learn from other countries? *Journal of Women, Politics and Policy, 30*(2), 301–334.

Hersch, J. (2009). Home production and wages: Evidence from the American Time Use Survey. *Review of Economics of the Household, 7*(2), 159–178.

Hewlett, S. (2002). *Creating a life: Professional women and the quest for children.* New York: Talk Miramax Books.

Heymann, J. (2000). *The widening gap: Why American working families are in jeopardy and what can be done about it.* New York: Basic Books.

Jandeska, K., & Kraimer, M. (2005). Women's perceptions of organizational culture, work attitudes, and role-modeling behaviors. *Journal of Managerial Issues, 18,* 461–478.

Karsten, M. (2006). Managerial women, minorities and stress: Causes and consequences. In M. Karsten (Ed.), *Gender, race and ethnicity in the workplace* (pp. 237–272). Westport, CT: Praeger.

Kempley, R. (1987). "Nuts." *Washington Post.* Retrieved on October 12, 2010, from http://www.washingtonpost.com/wp-srv/style/longterm/movies/videos/nutsrkempley_a0ca38.htm.

Landrine, H., & Russo, N. F. (Eds.). (2009). *Handbook of feminist psychology.* New York: Springer.

Lundberg-Love, P., & Marmion, S. (2006). *Intimate violence against women: When spouses, partners, or lovers attack.* Westport, CT: Praeger.

Marecek, J. (1978). Psychological disorders in women: Indices of role strain. In I. Frieze, J. Parsons, P. Johnson, D. Ruble, & G. Zellman (Eds.), *Women and sex roles: A social psychological perspective* (pp. 255–278). New York: Norton.

Marecek, J., & Kravertz, D. (1998). Putting policies into practice: Feminist therapy as feminist praxis. *Women and Therapy, 21,* 17–36.

McCann, J. (2001). *Stalking in children and adults: The primitive bond.* Washington, DC: American Psychological Association.

Milkie, M., Raley, S., & Bianchi, S. (2009). Taking on the second shift: Time allocations and time pressures of U.S. parents with preschoolers. *Social Forces, 88,* 487–517.

Moor, A. (2010). From victim to empowered survivor: Feminist therapy with survivors of rape and sexual assault. In M. Paludi (Ed.), *Feminism and women's rights worldwide* (Vol. 2, pp. 139–155). Santa Barbara, CA: Praeger.

Moor, A. (2011). Treating the sexually abused inner girl. In P. Lundberg-Love, K. Nadal, & M. Paludi (Eds.), *Women and mental disorders: Vol. 4. Treatment and research.* Santa Barbara, CA: Praeger.

Paludi, M. (2010, October). *The continuum of campus violence: Applying "Broken Windows Theory" to prevent and deal with campus violence.* Paper presented at the

U.S. Department of Education National Meeting on Alcohol, Drug Abuse and Violence Prevention in Higher Education, National Harbor, MD.

Paludi, M., & DeFour, D. C. (2010, September). "The test of a civilization is the way that it cares for its helpless members": Violence against older women. Paper presented at the New York Academy of Sciences and Pace University's Conference on Women, Power and Aging, New York City.

Paludi, M., & Denmark, F. (Eds.). (2011). *Victims of sexual assault and abuse: Resources and responses for individuals and families.* Santa Barbara, CA: Praeger.

Paludi, M., & Neidermeyer, P. (Eds.). (2008). *Work, life and family imbalance: How to level the playing field.* Westport, CT: Praeger.

Paludi, M., Vaccariello, R., Graham, T., Smith, M., Dicker, K., Kasprzak, H., & White, C. (2008). Work/life integration: Impact on women's careers, employment and family. In M. Paludi & P. Neidermeyer (Eds.), *Work, life and family imbalance: How to level the playing field* (pp. 21–36). Westport, CT: Praeger.

Pearce, D. (1978). The feminization of poverty: Women, work and welfare. *Urban and Social Change Review, 11,* 28–36.

Polakoff, E., & Gregory, D. (2002). Concepts on health: Women's struggle for wholeness in the midst of poverty. *Health Care for Women International, 23,* 835–845.

Pruis, T., & Janowsky, J. (2010). Assessment of body image in younger and older women. *Journal of Genetic Psychology, 137,* 225–238.

Russo, N. F. (1995). Women's mental health: Research agenda for the twenty-first century. In B. Brown, B. Kramer, P. Rieker, & C. Willie (Eds.), *Mental health, racism, and sexism* (pp. 373–396). Pittsburgh: University of Pittsburgh Press.

Russo, N. F., & Green, B. (1993). Women and mental health. In F. Denmark & M. Paludi (Eds.), *Psychology of women: A handbook of issues and theories* (pp. 379–436). Westport, CT: Praeger.

Russo, N. F., & Tartaro, J. (2008). Women and mental health. In F. Denmark & M. Paludi (Eds.). *Psychology of women: A handbook of issues and theories* (pp. 440–483). Westport, CT: Praeger.

Sachs-Ericsson, N., & Ciarlo, J. (2000). Gender, social roles and mental health: An epidemiological perspective. *Sex Roles: A Journal of Research, 43,* 339–362.

Showalter, E. (1985). *The female malady: Women, madness and English culture, 1830–1980.* New York: Penguin.

Sontag, S. (1979). The double standard of aging. In J. Williams (Ed.), *Psychology of women: Selected readings* (pp. 462–478). New York: Norton.

Strassel, K., Colgan, C., & Goodman, J. (2006). *Leaving women behind: Modern families, outdated laws.* New York: Rowman & Littlefield.

Thibos, M., Lavin-Loucks, D., & Martin, M. (2007). *The feminization of poverty: Empowering women.* Report prepared for the 2007 Joint Policy Forum on the Feminization of Poverty. Retrieved on October 12, 2010, from www.thewilliamsinstitute.org. United States Department of Labor, Bureau of Labor Statistics (2010). American Time Use Survey summary. Retrieved on October 12, 2010, from www.bls.gov/news.release/atus.nr0.htm.

Waits, B., & Lundberg-Love, P. (2008). The impact of campus violence on college students. In M. Paludi (Ed.), *Understanding and preventing campus violence* (pp. 51–70). Westport, CT: Praeger.

White, S. (2010). Extreme poverty and its impact on women's vulnerability to HIV transmission: A rights issue. *International Journal of Human Rights, 14,* 75–91.

Williams, J. (1983). *Psychology of women: Behavior in a biosocial context.* New York: Norton.

Worell, J. (1980). New directions in counseling women. *Personnel and Guidance Journal, 58,* 477–484.

Worell, J. (1990). Women: The psychological perspective. In M. Paludi & G. Steuernagel (Eds.), *Foundations for a feminist restructuring of the academic disciplines* (pp. 184–224). New York: Haworth.

Yonkers, K., & Hamilton, J. (1995). Psychotropic medications. In M. Weissman (Ed.), *Psychiatry update: Annual review* (Vol. 13, pp. 147–178). Washington, DC: American Psychiatric Press.

Chapter 1

Stranger and Acquaintance Rape

Cultural Constructions, Reactions, and Victim Experiences

Beth A. Watson, Kelly A. Kovack, and Maureen C. McHugh

RAPE: A PREVALENT AND PERSISTENT PROBLEM

Rape is a prevalent and persistent phenomenon that profoundly impacts the lives of women and girls in the United States. Cultural constructions of rape, sexuality, and gender roles contribute to the continued prevalence of rape and impact our response to rape victims. Changes in our conceptions of rape, modification of sexual scripts, and elimination of rape myths and victim-blaming responses may provide more effective interventions and lead to rape prevention.

Rape Is Prevalent

Somewhere in the United States a woman is raped every two minutes (Holmes & Holmes, 2002). The National Violence Against Women Survey found that 18% of women reported being victims of rape or attempted rape during their lifetime (Tjaden & Thoennes, 1998). The National College Health Risk Behavior Survey found that 20% of college students had been raped in their lifetime, and 15% had been raped since they were 13 years old (Brener, McMahon, Warren, & Douglas, 1999). Women in the United States have about a one in five chance of being raped.

Rape is prevalent worldwide (Brownmiller, 1975; Sanday, 1981), as are other forms of violence against women. One in three women worldwide have been victims of male violence (Heise, Ellsberg, & Gottemoeller, 1999). However, there are cultural variations in rape rates. The rates of rape are noticeably high in the United States relative to other industrialized cultures, resulting in some to label the United States a rape culture (e.g., Griffin, 1979; Scully & Marolla, 1998). Here we examine how cultural beliefs about rape and about male and female sexual interactions underlie the prevalence and persistence of rape in the United States. We consider how social beliefs and constructions of gender and sexuality impact our reactions to rape and influence victim's disclosures.

Rape Is Persistent

Although there is some variation in estimates depending on how rape is defined or measured and who the respondents are, a general conclusion is that the rate of rape in the United States has been relatively consistent at 15% prevalence over a woman's lifetime (Rozee & Koss, 2001). Rozee (2000) interprets the existing research on rape as documenting the persistence of rape. Rozee (2003) has critically examined rape prevention (avoidance) programs and advice, arguing that our current approaches are not only ineffective but also contribute to women's experience of fear and anxiety.

Rape Has a Profound Impact on Women's Lives

Rape has a significant negative impact on the physical and mental health of rape victims and survivors. In this chapter we review the clinically documented psychological effects of rape, some of which were originally identified as a "rape trauma syndrome" by Burgess and Holmstrom (1974) and are now often diagnosed as post-traumatic stress disorder (PTSD). We also examine other possible mental health outcomes of rape survivors and review current therapeutic intervention approaches to rape victims. Finally, we make some suggestions for approaches to rape prevention that address the issues of rape mythology and cultural construction of male and female sexuality.

SOCIOCULTURAL FACTORS AND CULTURAL CONSTRUCTIONS

Conceptions of Rape

Conceptions and definitions of rape and sexual assault have changed over time and remain contested; not everyone agrees about what constitutes rape. At one time rape was viewed as a crime against (the property) of men, that is, the fathers or husbands of the assaulted woman. Until the 1980s a man's rape of his wife was not legally a crime. Today, as a crime, rape is defined legally by each state. However, we are not discussing rape and sexual assault in legal terms but instead as an experience of women that impacts their lives and mental health. Although rape is the most often used term, the Centers for Disease Control and Prevention and the World Health Organization prefer the term "sexual violence," which includes sexually violating behaviors that may not meet legal thresholds as a crime but could have a detrimental impact on the individual's well-being. In this chapter we use the terms "rape" and "sexual assault" as interchangeable and subscribe to the definition given by the U.S. Department of Justice's Office of Violence Against Women: Sexual assault is "any type of sexual contact or behavior that occurs without the explicit consent of the recipient to the unwanted sexual activity."

Although individuals tend to believe that rape is perpetrated in dark alleys by a stranger and involves a weapon or a high level of injury, less than a third of all sexual assaults are committed by strangers. Acquaintance, date, and marital rape are more common than stranger rape. Current or former husbands, cohabitating partners or boyfriends, and dates commit 75% of rapes, according to the National Violence Against Women Survey. This discrepancy between our conception of rape and the reality of most rapes has created problems for victims of acquaintance, date, and marital rape. Rape has often remained hidden and has gone unreported when it occurs within normal dating relations (Koss, 1985) and in marriage (Russell, 1982). Some individuals, including police officers and school administrators, refer to stranger rapes as "real rapes," discounting the traumatic experience of acquaintance rape. Date, partner, and marital rapes require us to rethink our conceptions of rape but also challenge our ideas about what is acceptable sexual behavior within intimate relationships. Rozee (2000) argues that rape, and in particular date rape, is persistent because on some level forced and nonconsensual sex is permissible; she refers to it as "normative rape." These conceptions of rape impact societal reactions to rape victims and their recovery process, as discussed below.

We typically view girls and women as the targets or victims of rape and view men as the rapists. This is in fact accurate. The vast majority of rape cases involve male perpetrators and female victims. According to the Bureau of Justice Statistics National Crime Victimization Survey, 98% of the rapists were men, and 92% of the victims were girls or women. Throughout this chapter we will typically be using pronouns consistent with this type of rape, and our analysis examines how gender and gender roles contribute to the persistence of rape.

CULTURAL CONSTRUCTIONS OF RAPE

Rape as Power

Feminists have argued that rape is the result of an androcentric (male-oriented) culture that privileges male experience and desire. For example, Sanday (1981) analyzes rape as a function of cultural acceptance of male behavior, in particular aggression, and devaluation of feminine qualities in male-dominated societies. Rape is a reflection and a result of gender inequality, a tool and a consequence of gender oppression (Rozee, 2000). In this analysis, rape is in part the result of women having less power than men, and rape and other forms of violence against women are social practices that keep women powerless (Brownmiller, 1975).

Consistent with this analysis, women who have the least power in a society are the most vulnerable to rape. Among the most vulnerable individuals to be raped are immigrant women, especially the undocumented (Rozee & Van Boemel, 1995). Disabled women are three times more likely to be raped than able-bodied women (Holtzman, 1994). Rape is more commonly perpetrated against girls and young women; the vulnerability of young women and girls to rape can also be viewed in relation to their powerlessness. Older women are also vulnerable to rape, with potentially severe negative outcomes occurring. Furthermore, Logan, Evans, Stevenson, and Jordan (2005) found that women in lower socioeconomic status brackets were seven times more likely to have been victims of sexual violence than women with higher income levels. Goodman, Koss, and Russo (1979) reported that street crimes, including stranger rape, were more commonly perpetrated against poor and ethnic women. Wyatt (1992) similarly pointed out the vulnerability of Black women to stranger rape.

Although there do appear to be differences in rape rates related to ethnicity, the patterns of results are complex. Other studies do not confirm a higher rate of victimization of Black women (e.g., Koss & Dinero, 1989). The lifetime prevalence of rape is highest for White women, but it is believed that this is due to Black women and Latinas not coming forward as much or being blamed more frequently. Black women may not report a rape to institutions in a culture where their experience will not be seen as "real" rape because of their living situation; they must walk alone at night, take public transportation, and engage in other discouraged behaviors. Latinas have more traditional gender attitudes, including subscription to rape myths (discussed below) in comparison to European Americans and to African Americans (Lefley, Scott, Llabre, & Hicks, 1993). Asian women may be less likely to report a rape due to the fact that they may be less likely to recognize and label the occurrence as such (Mori, Bernat, Glenn, Selle, and Zarate, 1995). Race, culture, class, age, and sexual orientation affect every aspect of rape including recovery from the sexual violence experience (Paludi, 1999). Research by Koss, Heise, and Russo (1994) indicates that male violence against women crosses all racial, ethnic, socioeconomic, age, and sexual orientation boundaries.

CULTURAL ATTITUDES RELATED TO REACTIONS TO RAPE VICTIMS

Feminist authors have argued that an understanding of the experience of rape requires an analysis of the cultural context in which rape is persistently committed. Feminist theory stresses that rape is both socially produced and socially legitimized. Our conceptions of rape and our cultural attitudes toward male and female sexuality may contribute to the prevalence of rape and definitely impacts our reactions to rapists and victims. Cultural attitudes toward women, gender, sexuality, and aggression underlie our criminal justice system and influence the treatment that victims receive in a wide range of agencies and settings. Rozee (2000) argues that the persistence and prevalence of rape may best be explained by examining our cultural constructions and attitudes toward rape. We examine how gender roles, conceptions of male and female sexuality, sexual scripts for sexual interactions, conceptions and misconceptions about rape, and victim blame contribute to the persistence of rape and negatively impact our reactions to rape victims.

Sexual Scripts

Sexual scripts are theorized to have an impact on individuals' sexual behavior, including rape. Scripts are cognitive characterizations of a particular sequence of events, such as going out on a first date or going to a movie (Simon & Gagnon, 1984, 1986). Scripts include expectations, roles, and norms for interactions in different contexts. The "traditional" sexual script for heterosexual interactions positions men as initiators of sexual activity and women as the reactors or "gatekeepers," responsible for controlling the pace (Brooks, 1995; Tiefer, 1995). The traditional sexual script positions men and women as adversaries (Castaneda & Burns-Glover, 2004), which sets the stage for coerced sex and rape. In the script, sexual interactions are like a competitive game in which men use multiple strategies to persuade women to engage in sex and women use multiple strategies to avoid sexual intercourse.

Sexual scripts may play a key role in how people understand and enact sexual interactions. That is, forced sexual activity may not be labeled as rape because it does not fit with an individual's rape script. In a study conducted by Littleton and Axsom (2003), when participants described a rape script and a seduction script, both scripts tended to involve the use of manipulative tactics on the part of the man to obtain sex and to involve women engaging in sexual activity that they did not want. This overlap in manipulative tactics in sexual scripts may lead to more incidences of rape or also to individuals not reporting a rape. Kahn and his colleagues (Kahn, Mathie, & Torglar, 1994) examined differences in scripts of acknowledged and unacknowledged rape victims, that is, women who had an experience that fits the definition of rape but do not label the experience as rape. Unacknowledged rape victims had a rape script that involved a violent attack by a stranger, whereas acknowledged rape victims had scripts that included acquaintance rape. This documents our suspicion that in our culture, given our scripts for rape and our attitudes toward male sexuality, individuals may not view coerced or forced sex as a crime. In a related study where undergraduates responded to a sexual situation/script, Lewin (1985) found that half of women student respondents felt that unwanted intercourse obtained through pressure was acceptable behavior and even thought that the acquaintance rapist/man might fall in love with them. This research confirms Rozee's (2000) contention that women construe acquaintance rape—that is, unwanted sexual intercourse performed under pressure—as normative. Similarly, college men may not identify acquaintance rape as rape. Lott (1994) found that a majority of young men thought that it was acceptable to force sex on a woman if they had been dating a long time or if they were planning to marry. Koss, Leonard, Beezley, & Oros (1985) reported that 12% of their male respondents reported engaging in sexual behavior that qualified as rape, but the respondents said that it was definitely not rape. Krahe (1991) reports that police officers similarly adopt a traditional view of male and female sexual interaction. Their rape script involved violent force, a stranger assailant, and an outdoor context. The police officers viewed acquaintance rape that involved low levels of force as dubious.

These and other related studies indicate that sexist attitudes and/or traditional gender roles—beliefs about appropriate roles and behaviors for men and women, including intimate and sexual relationships—impact our constructions of rape and our reactions to rape victims. Sexual scripts are one mechanism by which individuals learn and adopt gender roles in their intimate and sexual interactions. To the extent that sexual scripts incorporate normative social practices and traditional gender roles, sexual scripts maintain the status quo, including the subordination of women and the sexual double standard.

The Sexual Double Standard

The sexual double standard refers to the acceptance of different standards used to evaluate the sexual behavior of men and women. The sexual double standard is a set of standards under which men are rewarded for engaging in sexual experiences, whereas women are derogated or chastised for similar sexual experiences. The sexual double standard perpetuates traditional gender role stereotypes. According to Lees (1986), boys can control girls' reputations and are better able to pressure them into relationships because girls fear being labeled as promiscuous. This also impacts women's ability to negotiate safer sex practices, such as the use of condoms (Holland, Ramazanoglu, Scott, Sharpe, & Thomson, 1991). Although some research suggests a decline of the sexual double standard as an individually held attitude, other more qualitative research documents sexual double standard as a social practice (Crawford & Popp, 2003). For example, McHugh, Watson, and Sullivan (2009) have demonstrated the phenomenon of slut bashing as a social practice that is based on and promotes a sexual double standard.

One unfortunate consequence of the sexual double standard is miscommunication. In a study conducted by Muehlenhard (1988), men reportedly attempted to analyze women's behaviors rather than attempt discussion of sexual desires. The study found that men are more likely to interpret friendly behaviors as signals that the other person is interested in sex, and men tended to rate a woman as somewhat wanting sex, even if she had said "no" multiple times or forcefully attempted to stop the man. Men may believe that a woman is only saying "no" because she is acting according to the sexual double standard. Unless in relationships, women cannot indicate that they want to engage in sex, so women may engage in token refusal. According to this script, not only can a man ignore a girl's refusal because it is token, but he should ignore her refusal because a man who stops when a woman says no is not sufficiently masculine. Although this study did find that some women engaged in token resistance, it was much more frequent that the men misinterpreted the woman's resistance as token. Krahe and colleagues (2000) found a strong link between men's beliefs that women engage in token resistance and reported aggression against female partners. Thus, it should be stressed here that no woman should engage in token resistance, as the few incidences of genuine token resistance perpetuate this idea for men. Additionally, the myth of token resistance is further perpetuated by pornography, jokes, and movies in our society, which lead to the development of rape myths.

Rape Myths

The prevalence and persistence of rape have frequently been tied to the operation of rape myths in our culture. Rape myths are stereotypical, prejudicial, and invalid ideas about rape that are disadvantageous to women. The basic premise of rape myths include the notion that real rapes are those that conform to a rape sexual script in which a stranger uses a weapon or extreme force to engage in sexual intercourse with a resisting and innocent woman. Rape myths are problematic not only because they are not accurate but also because they serve several functions that are harmful to rape victims. These descriptive and prescriptive beliefs about the causes, context, consequences, perpetrators, and victims of rape serve to deny, trivialize, or justify sexual violence exerted by men against women (Bohner, Siebler, & Schmelcher, 2006).

Burt (1998) illuminated multiple components of rape myths. One rape myth perspective is that nothing happened, or rape did not occur. This perspective includes the position that women make up or exaggerate accounts of rape. Another rape myth often argues that no harm was done; this myth is frequently applied to sexually experienced women, suggesting that having nonconsensual sex with a virgin is the only foul. The most commonly applied myths concern women's participation in the assault in the form of provocation, precipitation, or pleasure. These victim-blaming rape myths are based on the sexual scripts and sexual double standards already discussed. Sexual behavior of men is acceptable, as they have high uncontrollable sex drives and cannot control themselves when provoked by women. Women, however, are charged with restraining themselves and men from sexual interactions. Thus, if sex occurred, the women was responsible. Other aspects of our rape myths include conceptions as rapists as deviant men who lack access to sexual partners. Rape myths are reinforced by jokes; in the media, both in the mainstream films and television; and in pornography (Burt, 1998; Malamuth, 1984).

In Burt's (1998) analysis, rape myths operate to maintain male advantage in a male-dominant culture. Women live with the fear of rape and modify their behavior to avoid rape. Women are held responsible for the prevention of their own rape and are viewed as provoking it or enjoying it if they are not successful. Based on rape myths, victims are blamed by others and frequently blame themselves. Acquaintance rape is discounted and hidden, and victim blame is especially likely for victims who had been drinking and/or who were raped at parties or in a residence.

There is evidence that, as theorized, rape myth acceptance impacts our interactions and our reactions to rape victims. For example, rapists subscribe to rape myths more than nonraping men, and men subscribe to rape myths more than women. Individuals who subscribe to rape myths are more prone to victim blaming and are less likely to convict rapists in jury studies. Most importantly, some researchers have provided evidence that rape myth acceptance in men is associated with rape proclivity (Malamuth & Check, 1985). Chapleau and Oswald (2010) found that individuals who associated power and sex tended to also accept rape myths more frequently than others, which leads to a greater likelihood of these individuals becoming perpetrators.

Victim Blame

As indicated by this analysis, rape myths incorporate a victim-blaming perspective on rape. Victims are viewed as having precipitated, provoked, and/or enjoyed the rape experience, or at the very least they did not protect themselves or resist sufficiently. Victim blaming occurs when we hold victims responsible for their own fate. In regional or national cases of rape accusations, victims are frequently portrayed in the media as lying to receive attention or financial resources.

Psychologists have documented the existence of victim blaming and have proposed reasons for the victim-blaming responses. One model of victim blaming theorized by Lerner (1980) is that victim blaming allows us to retain our belief in a just world, a world where good things happen to good people. When apparently good individuals experience a negative event or fate, this threatens our belief in a just world. One way to restore a belief in a just world is to find ways in which the victim is at fault. A second model, an attributional approach, argues that we try to find aspects of the victim to blame so that we do not have to consider having the same fate occur to us. While victim blaming is a general phenomena that occurs in varied situations, much of the blaming research has focused on the blame attributed to women victims of male violence.

Victim-blaming reactions from others have been referred to as secondary victimization (Campbell & Raja, 1999), and research indicates that secondary victimization is a common experience of rape victims (Ulman, 2010). Blaming responses take one of two forms, according to Ulman (2010). Overt blaming involves explicit statements such as "it was your fault." Implicit blaming typically occurs by questioning the victim about her activities, her decisions, etc. Research indicates that victims are blamed by both informal and formal networks. Agency personnel such as police, physicians, pastors, and psychologists who are supposed to provide assistance or support to rape victims frequently engage in victim-blaming responses (Ulman, 2010). Unfortunately, family, friends, and colleagues also demonstrate similar victim blaming tendencies.

Victim blaming discourages women from reporting their sexual assault to the criminal justice system. Rape is the most underreported crime. Failure to report rape undermines the potential of the police and criminal justice system to prevent rape. We underestimate the prevalence of rape when victims decide not to disclose the experience. Ironically, the prevalence rates should counteract our tendency to blame victims. When rape is a normative experience, the tendency should be to look for larger, more structural explanations. Blaming individuals for common events violates common sense.

Rape survivors often remain silent about their experience. They may not report the rape to authorities or even disclose it to their friends and families. Individuals from both formal and informal networks of support often react to victims negatively. At the minimum, one-fourth and as many as three-fourths of survivors receive negative social reactions from someone in their support networks (Campbell et al., 2001). Ahrens (2006) interviewed victims who were silent following an initial disclosure to examine the reasons for victims' silence. She demonstrated that the negative reactions of others, including blaming and doubting, contribute to that silence. All of the victims reported insensitive and blaming reactions. Ahrens reports that negative reactions received from friends and families reinforced victims' feelings of self-blame, and reactions from professionals led to victims questioning the advisability of disclosure.

Blaming was one of the negative unsupportive or upsetting reactions that victims reported to Ingram, Betz, Mindes, Schmitt, Smith (2001); the other negative reactions were distancing, minimizing, and bumbling. Unsupportive social interactions impacted the victims' experience of psychological symptoms. Negative reactions from family members, such as expressing shame, overreacting, focusing on their own anger or frustration, or trying to control the behavior of the victim, negatively impact the victim's recovery outcomes (Filipas & Ullman, 2001).

THE NEGATIVE IMPACT OF RAPE ON WOMEN'S MENTAL HEALTH

Physical Health Impact

Rape results in a range of negative outcomes for victims. Many rape victims have multiple physical health outcomes including bruising, internal damage and infections, and other injuries. Victims may contract a sexually transmitted infection, and about 5% of rapes result in pregnancy. The physical consequences of rape are most likely underestimated, as many victims do not seek medical attention, and medical personnel do not always inquire about the source of injuries treated (Goodman et al., 1979). Some rape victims, even those who do not acknowledge or label their negative sexual experience as rape, subsequently have somatic symptoms including headaches, fatigue, disturbances in sleep and appetite, and irritability. In a longitudinal study, Koss and Harvey (1991) documented increased visits to the physician in the second year following a sexual assault. The distinction between physical and mental health effects is not clear-cut. Physical symptoms may be caused by severe psychological distress and may be genuinely experienced in a physical sense. Other somatic symptoms may result from increased attention to physical symptoms, and complaints may be more noticeable as the victim's sense of personal threat is heightened.

Mental Health Effects

Rape victims suffer both immediate and longer-term mental health effects (Goodman et al., 1979). Fear and anxiety predominate initially. During and after a sexual assault, a survivor's reaction may include intense fear, helplessness, or horror. Other reactions following the event include sudden shifts in mood or moodiness, flashbacks, and relationship difficulty (American Psychological Association, 2010). She may also experience hyperarousal, including such symptoms as sleep problems, irritability, an exaggerated startle response, hypervigilance, and difficulty concentrating. A survivor may also show an avoidance of stimuli associated with the assault, interpersonal and emotional numbness, detachment or lack of interest, diminished expectations about her future, and difficulty recalling important aspects of the trauma. Initial experiences of fear, shock, and confusion may decrease after several months, but sometimes these reactions reappear years later. About one-fourth of rape victims have severe and extended symptoms beyond this initial reaction.

Sexually assaulted women may develop symptoms of anxiety disorders, depression, suicidality, eating disorders, dissociative disorders, and substance use. By definition, trauma consists of the "emotional response following a terrible event" (American Psychological Association, 2010). Survivors may also feel as if the event is being reexperienced in various ways, including recurrent and distressing dreams or memories of the event, feeling or acting as if the assault is happening again, and intense emotional and physiological reactivity when exposed to inner or external cues associated with the assault.

These clusters of symptoms that may comprise the survivor's reaction are characteristics required for a formal diagnosis of post-traumatic stress disorder (PTSD) or acute stress disorder according to the *DSM-IV-TR* (American Psychiatric Association, 2000). Woman develop PTSD approximately twice as often as males and are at higher risk for PTSD if another traumatic event happens after having previously experienced a violent assault such as rape (Breslau & Anthony, 2007). Survivors of sexual assault and other traumatic events often do not develop symptoms that fit neatly into the categories of one disorder or another and may experience a combination of symptoms that can span across diagnostic categories and would be seen as subclinical, or not meeting full criteria for a specific disorder. Although sexual assaults fit the general perception of an event that is traumatic, each woman may have a different response following the assault. Her reaction may be the result of a range of factors such as different background experiences, assault characteristics, and responses of health care providers, law enforcement, and others in her support system. For example, experiencing and coping with victimization in isolation is connected to severity of symptoms, and better recovery is tied to the availability of positive social support. The acceptance of rape myths by family friends and professionals can impede recovery as discussed.

Along with a sense of foreshortened future, other signs of hopelessness and feelings of worthlessness may surface in the aftermath of a sexual assault. Clinical levels of depression may develop in accordance with the rape survivor's shattered view of the world. Her assumptions, which may or may not have previously included the belief in a just world, have been deeply and personally challenged (Janoff-Bulman, 1992, pp. 78–81). A survivor who has experienced rape or another traumatic event in the past may develop a strong belief in her lack of control over the events in her life. A sexual assault may strip a woman of her hope and aspirations toward the future. However, Fine (1983) has argued that this may be a class bias in psychological theory, since many women, especially working-class and poor women, did not experience a sense of control prior to the assault.

The rape victim may develop negative feelings toward herself due to the blame and guilt that social messages tend to elicit around sexual violence. In addition to the blame-saturated messages that surround women, after gathering personal evidence about her own vulnerability a rape survivor may have increasing difficulty staving off the feelings of helplessness that may have been present prior to the rape. The survivor may also lose confidence in others, developing doubts that there are good people out there in the world. She may feel that she is becoming hostile or outraged at the wrongdoings of others and injustices seen in the world and may feel even more helpless. This sense that the world is spinning out of control coupled with despair and conflicting feelings of anger and pain may lead to the development of symptoms that would be considered to be characteristic of depression. Along with feelings of depression, suicidal ideation and attempts may occur in some survivors (Campbell, Dworkin, & Cabral, 2009).

Survivors of rape may also develop symptoms that are not typically associated with PTSD or depression. They may exhibit symptoms of other anxiety disorders, such as phobias or intense fears of specific stimuli, panic attacks, agoraphobia or fear of leaving home, and generalized anxiety or pervasive worrying. Substance use, including binge drinking, marijuana use, and illicit drug use, has been shown to increase following incapacitated, forcible, or drug/alcohol-facilitated rape experiences (Campbell, Dworkin, & Cabral, 2009; McCauley, Ruggeiro, Resnick, & Kilpatrick, 2010). Rape victims are more likely to be diagnosed with a substance dependence than are nonvictims even years after the assault (Goodman et al. 1979). Survivors of sexual assault have shown patterns of increased cigarette smoking as well.

Victims of sexual assault may experience a range of sexual dysfunctions. Some victims report arousal dysfunction, decreased sexual interest, and/or fear of sex. Other psychological effects of date rape and stranger rape may include various levels of guilt, shame, and self-blame (Frieze, 2005; Koss, 2000). These reactions have been connected to cultural myths about rape, including victim blaming. Rape victims frequently demonstrate social withdrawal, lowered sociability, and lowered self-esteem. Even when they continue interacting socially, some victims report less enjoyment and pleasure in life.

PERSONAL GROWTH AND COPING FOLLOWING RAPE

In addition to the expected development of pathology in response to a traumatic event such as rape, some survivors also report positive outcomes in the aftermath of their assault. Post-traumatic growth (PTG) is a concept that has fairly recently gained attention in the trauma literature in conjunction with the positive psychology movement. PTG refers to positive changes following a traumatic event, regardless of the negative changes that also occurred. PTG also has been referred to as resilience, thriving, benefit finding, stress-related growth, adversarial growth, optimism, and positive illusions (Calhoun & Tedeschi, 1998; Folkman, 2008; Taylor & Armor, 1996). These terms found throughout the trauma literature reflect various attempts to find a word for the very meaningful outcomes that develop as a result of the existential challenge that follows facing one's mortality or serious changes to one's life (Yalom & Lieberman, 1991). The components of PTG often include changes in one's sense of personal strength, improved relationships with others, increased compassion for others, the development of personal life philosophies or spirituality, appreciation of life, reorganization of priorities, recognition of new possibilities or paths for one's life, affect regulation, self-understanding, belongingness, optimism, wisdom and skills, honesty and reliability, and acceptance.

Beyond a lack of psychopathology or diagnosable symptoms of distress, PTG encompasses the essence of a survivor in developing new outlooks and personal meaning after such a physically and emotionally traumatic event such as date rape or stranger rape. Distress and growth often accompany one another in survivors' experiences. The exact relationship between PTSD and the potential for PTG is unknown at this time. In some studies PTG is associated with lower rates of PTSD, whereas in other studies PTG is associated with higher levels of PTSD or depression (Calhoun & Tedeschi, 1998; Kleim & Ehlers, 2009). Estimated prevalence rates for PTG also greatly vary, ranging from 3% to 98% (Linley & Joseph, 2004). In acknowledging positive changes that some victims experience after a rape, there is no denial of the horrific experience that the survivor endured. Increasingly researchers stress the value in adopting a model of coping following a trauma such as rape that considers positive changes, negative changes, and no change in various dimensions of life (Calhoun & Tedeschi, 1998).

It can be a puzzling phenomenon that someone would find benefits in having persevered through a trauma. On the other hand, some therapists have taken positive psychology concepts and forced them onto survivors, suggesting that they look at the bright side, that they are lucky to be alive, and other such well-meant but unsupportive or detrimental comments. One key aspect in understanding the idea of PTG is that this does not encourage individuals to label a traumatic event as positive. Instead, positive aspects may be found in the rape survivor's incredible strength that may have emerged or developed in working through the assault. It is important not to encourage her to "grin and bear it," as society has long placed women in a position of facing hardships without complaint. Women at times have been seen as weak when they expressed emotional distress. Women also consistently report more positive changes or PTG, even when accompanied by substantial amounts of distress (Vishnevsky et al., 2010).

It is extremely important to be mindful of the distress that a survivor has endured and to avoid providing unsupportive social reactions by encouraging the survivor to "see the bright side" or focus solely on positive things, such as feeling "lucky to be alive." It is also extremely encouraging that the distress that survivors may experience is eventually accompanied by positive changes, personal growth, and recovery resulting from the role they enact as survivors in the face of adversity (Park & Helgeson, 2006). Not all survivors experience PTG, and they should not be pressured or expected to be satisfied with the horrific event. Those who report PTG may have different experiences during and after the trauma that allow them to develop an appreciation for themselves, others, and life in general that develops in the aftermath of the trauma. Regardless of this appreciation, survivors do not report being content that the event itself occurred.

The field of psychology has traditionally emphasized the reduction of distress, but some distress is natural after experiencing a sexual assault. Distress can be seen as adaptive in some situations if it helps to mobilize and activate coping resources after a crisis such as a rape (Kleim & Ehlers, 2009). One idea that is thought to serve a short-term protective function is that of positive illusions. Although mental health professionals generally suggest that those in close contact with reality have better outcomes, traumatic events may pose an exception to the rule, as a sexual assault is not expected to occur. It also appears that people who report more life satisfaction tend to show some positively distorted perceptions in their everyday lives (Taylor & Armor, 1996). In the context of rape, positive illusions following the assault may serve a short-term function in helping a survivor to cope with the overwhelming trauma she has experienced, facilitating the search for meaning in her experience, regaining a sense of master, and restoring a positive sense of self (Taylor & Armor, 1996). As some researchers have found positive changes similar to PTG reported very soon after sexual assault, initial reports of growth may be a form of positive illusion that sets the trajectory for later growth (Folkman, 2008; Taylor & Armor, 1996).

In the coping literature, women regularly are shown to engage in coping strategies associated with distress. These strategies typically are labeled as maladaptive, as researchers exhibit a tendency to label coping strategies broadly as adaptive or maladaptive (Littleton, Horsley, John, & Nelson, 2007). A paradox is seen in women reporting more PTG while also reporting that they engage in coping strategies labeled as maladaptive due to their association with distress.

Coping with a trauma such as rape presents several challenges. The survivor's methods of coping may include tasks such as processing the information and implications of the painful event, rebuilding her assumptions, and dealing with others (Janoff-Bulman, 1992). These processes are not the only coping challenges that a survivor faces, and she may be faced with many different tasks at once. Shock and denial, somewhat natural responses or defenses when a seemingly overwhelming challenge arises, eventually transition into an understanding of what it is that has happened. An unnatural event such as rape, though regrettably common, does not fit naturally into one's state of mind. Even if a rape or other trauma has occurred before, each encounter with a horrible experience poses some unique challenges. The information must be incorporated into the existing knowledge base and beliefs. Beliefs then must sometimes be altered or rebuilt. In a moment of violence, beliefs that may have existed for a woman's lifetime or that have certainly existed longer than the rape experience lasts can be shattered without regard to how true they may seem. Because a trauma is unexpected and horrific, beliefs that were solid may have no meaning. A new paradigm for approaching life begins to form, incorporating this new experience into the rubble of a shattered belief system. In addition to rebuilding her life from the inside out, dealing with others is another challenge. The victim may encounter others' supportive and unsupportive reactions in their various roles and responsibilities, interactions with members of the legal and health care systems, and society as a whole.

INTERVENTIONS WITH RAPE VICTIMS

In general, victims tend to rate their experiences with mental health professionals as positive and characterize their help as useful and supportive (Campbell et al., 2001). Victims who had difficulty obtaining services or experienced victim blaming from the legal and medical system had high PTSD symptomatology, while those who obtained mental health services had lower PTSD rates, suggesting benefits to therapy. This also indicates the importance of therapists and counselors unlearning victim-blaming myths and perspectives. Unfortunately, therapy is not necessarily available to all victims of rape, and some counselors continue to perpetrate victim blaming and other nonsupportive reactions. The majority of rape victims who seek services are Caucasian and have health insurance (Campbell et al. 2001).

There are many different types of treatments available for rape victims, just as there are for anyone struggling with depression, anxiety, or any other mental health problems. However, rape victims have a special need that other individuals may not need to consider: therapy for rape victims needs to provide accurate information about rape, societal blame, and self-blame. Although mental health is still somewhat stigmatized in our society, it is much less likely for an individual suffering from schizophrenia to be blamed than it is for an individual who has survived rape. Therapy for rape victims also needs to promote healthy relationships and social support, as these are both factors that can help individuals in the recovery process. Many survivors receive negative social reactions from their informal network, and survivors are also likely to receive negative reactions from formal support providers (Ahrens, 2006; Ulman, 2010). Therapists must accept the woman's reality about the rape, or else women may experience the same revictimization in therapy that they have been experiencing in the criminal justice system and society at large. Therapy can provide rape victims with a safe place to tell their story without a negative or blaming reaction.

One consideration is that women who have been raped may want to begin therapy with a feminist therapist. Feminist therapists emphasize the sociocultural context of rape and challenge victim-blaming perspectives. When deciding on a therapist, an individual can ask the therapist about her positions on rape in our society and on victim blaming in order to find a therapist who fits well with the individual and also will not revictimize but instead will empower the individual. Therapy for survivors of rape should be empowering. According to Lamb (1996), one problem with this is that there are enough stories of victims who overcome their victimization to demoralize those who do not or cannot. The overarching question, then, is should we hold victims responsible for their reactions to trauma and symptoms? On the one hand, yes, because it gives them agency and power, but on the other hand, no, because it is blaming the victim even more. It is a balancing act at times in therapy, but the most important thing that we can stress to any individual considering therapy is to trust your instincts. If you do not feel comfortable with your therapist or you believe that the therapist is hurting you more than helping you, you do not have to stay. There are many therapists in the world, and it is crucial to your recovery that you choose someone with whom you feel comfortable.

In addition to traditional outpatient mental health offices, a survivor of rape may also consider receiving help through a rape crisis center. Only 3% to 21% of rape victims reportedly utilize rape crisis centers. This is unfortunate, as the centers tend to have a strong feminist and/or empowerment theoretical orientation. Edmond (2006) found that approximately 70% of rape crisis centers use cognitive-behaviorist therapy methods in combination with these other more feminist methods. Studies have found significant reductions in distress levels and self-blame over time and increases in social support, self-efficacy, and sense of control when individuals went to a rape crisis center.

Obviously, not all of the entire recovery process will occur during therapy sessions but also occurs while talking to friends or family members. According to Tyra (1993), these nontherapist supports should be concerned and available, give the individual time and a place to vent, help remind the individual that she is not to blame, give information about other resources and therapists (if the individual has not already sought out these resources herself), and help identify other emotionally supportive people in the victim's life. According to Ulman (2010), when survivors felt validated and believed by others, their self-blame feelings tended to diminish. Friends are especially likely to be the recipient of rape disclosure, and victims find them to be the most helpful source of support (Ahrens et al., 2006; Ulman, 2010). Supportive friends have a positive impact on the victim's recovery.

PREVENTION

Many current rape prevention programs focus primarily on what women can do to avoid rape. For example, women are advised to not walk alone or frequent certain locations. This approach to prevention confirms the rape myth perspective that rape is the result of what women do and do not do. These programs also convey the notion that men are inherently sexual, irresponsible, and uncontrollable. As Rozee (2003) points out, these programs do not prevent rape but merely support rape myths and sexual scripts. A multivariate study by Norris and Kaniasty (1992) found that precautionary behaviors of women had no preventive impact on the subsequent occurrence of crime. More importantly, this form of rape prevention contributes to women's fear and anxiety. The anxiety that women feel limits their movement and activity. Fear of rape keeps women in their place: at home, following social conventions.

Alternative approaches to rape prevention have been developed as a result of feminist activism starting in the 1970s. Rape crisis centers, universities, and community organizations have developed rape prevention and education programs focused on changing attitudes and empowering women. Commonly, such programs challenge rape myths and other rape-supportive attitudes and provide information on rape to a range of audiences. Evaluation of such programs indicates a small degree of attitude change that is short term (Ahrens et al., 2008). In a comprehensive review of rape education programs, Lonsway (1996) found that only half of the programs decreased rape-supportive attitudes, and attitude change was not sustained in the long term. More effective programs were ones that were interactive multiple-session programs facilitated by professional educators (Anderson & Whiston, 2005). Unfortunately, programs have not yet demonstrated any effectiveness in reducing rape (Anderson & Whiston, 2005; Rozee & Koss, 2001; Campbell & Wasco, 2005). However, attitude change programs may impact the type of reaction that rape victims receive from family, friends, and community members.

Sexual violence is often hidden or dismissed or seen as normative behavior. Prevention begins with recognizing the prevalence of rape and acknowledging the profound impact that rape has on the lives of victims and on the lives of all girls and women. Prevention must involve changing our sexual scripts, challenging the sexual double standard, and criticizing rape myths. When we support rape victims rather than blame them, we can encourage them to talk about their experiences. Even as we attempt to repair the damage at the individual level, we must shift our focus to challenging the sexual double standard, sexual scripts, and rape myths and changing our cultural constructions of gender, sexuality, intimate relationships, and equality. We need to address the social institutions and social practices that incorporate and maintain male dominance and gender inequality. Some programs attempt to improve communication between sexual partners and between men and women more generally. Most importantly, rape prevention ultimately needs to address and modify the sexually aggressive behavior of men. From a feminist perspective, rape prevention includes critical examination and the challenge of gender roles and gender inequality. Feminist efforts to change the sociocultural conditions are essential. In encouraging us, Rozee (2000) joins Charlotte Bunch (1997, p. 44), who states that "There is nothing immutable about the violent oppression of women and girls. It is a construct of power, as was apartheid, and one that can be changed."

REFERENCES

Ahrens, C. E. (2006). Being silenced: The impact of negative social reactions on the disclosure of rape. *American Journal of Community Psychology, 38,* 263–274.

Ahrens, C. E., Dean, K., Rozee, P. D., & McKenzie, M. (2008). Understanding and preventing rape. In F. L. Denmark & M. A. Paludi (Eds.), *Psychology of women: A handbook of issues and theories* (2nd ed., pp. 509–554). Westport, CT: Praeger.

American Psychiatric Association. (2000). *Diagnostic and Statistical Manual of Mental Disorders* (4th ed.). Washington, DC: American Psychiatric Association.

American Psychological Association. (2010). *Trauma.* Retrieved on February 2, 2011, from http://www.apa.org/topics/trauma/index.aspx.

Amstadter, A. B., Resnick, H. S., Nugent, N. R., Acierno, R., Rheingold, A. A., Minhinnett, R., et al. (2009). Longitudinal trajectories of cigarette smoking following rape. *Journal of Traumatic Stress, 22,* 113–121.

Anderson, I., & Doherty, K. (2008). *Accounting for rape: Psychology, feminism, and disclosure analysis in the study of sexual violence.* New York: Routledge.

Anderson, L. A., & Whiston, S. C. (2005). Sexual assault education programs: A meta-analytic examination of their effectiveness. *Psychology of Women Quarterly, 29,* 374–388.

Bohner, G., Siebler, F., & Schmelcher, J. (2006). Social norms and the likelihood of raping: Perceived rape myth acceptance of others affects men's rape proclivity. *Personality and Social Psychology Bulletin, 32,* 286–297.

Brener, N. D., McMahon, P. M., Warren, C. W., & Douglas, K. A. (1999). Forced sexual intercourse and associated risk behaviors among female college students in the United States. *Journal of Counseling and Clinical Psychology, 67,* 252–259.

Breslau, N. (2009). The epidemiology of trauma, PTSD, and other posttrauma disorders. *Trauma, Violence, & Abuse, 10,* 198–210.

Breslau, N., & Anthony, J. C. (2007). Gender differences in the sensitivity to post-traumatic stress disorder: An epidemiological study of urban young adults. *Journal of Abnormal Psychology, 116,* 607–611.

Brooks, G. (1995). Challenging dominant discourses of male heterosexuality: The clinical implications of new voices about male sexuality. In P. Kleinplatz (Ed.), *New directions in sex therapy: Innovations and alternatives* (pp. 50–68). Philadelphia: Brunner-Routledge.

Brownmiller, S. (1975). *Against our will: Men, women and rape.* New York: Simon & Schuster.

Bunch, C. (1997). The intolerable status quo: Violence against women and girls. In Nations Children Fund (Ed.), *The progress of nations* (pp 41–49). New York: UNICEF.

Burgess, A., & Holmstrom, L. (1974). Rape trauma syndrome. *American Journal of Psychiatry, 131,* 981–986.

Burt, M. (1998). Rape myths. In M. E. Oden & J. Clay-Warner (Eds.), *Confronting rape and sexual assault* (pp. 129–144). Wilmington, DE: Scholarly Resources.

Calhoun, L. G., & Tedeschi, R. G. (1998). Beyond recovery from trauma: Implications for clinical practice. *Journal of Social Issues, 54,* 357–371.

Campbell, R., Ahrens, C. E., Sefl, T., Wasco, S. M., & Barnes, H. E. (2001). Social reactions to rape victims: Healing and hurtful effects on psychological and physical health outcomes. *Violence and Victims, 16,* 287–302.

Campbell, R., Dworkin, E., & Cabral, G. (2009). An ecological model of the impact of sexual assault on women's mental health. *Trauma, Violence, & Abuse, 10,* 225–246.

Campbell, R., & Raja, S. (1999). Secondary victimization of rape victims: Insights from mental health professionals who treat survivors of violence. *Violence and Victims, 14,* 261–275.

Campbell, R., & Wasco, S. (2005). Understanding rape and sexual assault: 20 years of progress and future directions. *Journal of Interpersonal Violence, 16,* 1239–1259.

Castaneda, D., & Burns-Glover, A. (2004). Gender, sexuality and close relationships. In M. Paludi (Ed.), *Praeger guide to the psychology of gender* (pp. 69–91). Westport, CT: Praeger.

Chapleau, K. M., & Oswald, D. L. (2010). Power, sex, and rape myth acceptance: Testing two models of rape proclivity. *Journal of Sex Research, 47,* 66–78.

Crawford, M., & Popp, D. (2003). Sexual double standards: A review and methodological critique of two decades of research. *Journal of Sex Research, 40,* 13–26.

Edmond, T. (2006, February). *Theoretical and intervention preferences of service providers addressing violence against women: A national survey*. Presented at Council of Social Work Education Conference, Chicago, IL.

Filipas, H. H., & Ullman, S. E. (2001). Social reactions to sexual assault victims from various support sources. *Violence and Victims, 16,* 673–692.

Fine, M. (1983). Coping with rape: Critical perspectives on consciousness. *Imagination, Cognition and Personality, 3,* 249–264.

Folkman, S. (2008). The case for positive emotions in the stress process. *Anxiety, Stress, & Coping, 21,* 3–14.

Frieze, I. H. (2005). *Hurting the one you love: Violence in relationships.* Belmont, CA: Thomson Wadsworth.

Gagnon, J., & Simon, W. (1973). *Sexual conduct: The social sources of human sexuality.* Chicago: Aldine.

Gilbert, P. R., & Eby, K. K. (Eds.). (2003). *Violence and gender: An interdisciplinary reader.* Upper Saddle River, NJ: Pearson/Prentice Hall.

Goodman, L. A., Koss, M. P., & Russo, N. F. (1979). Violence against women: Physical and mental health effects. In S. Griffin (Ed.), *Rape: The politics of consciousness.* San Francisco: Harper & Row.

Griffin, S. (1979). *Rape: The politics of consciousness.* San Francisco: Harper & Row.

Heise, L., Ellsberg, M., & Gottemoeller, M. (1999). Ending violence against women. *Population Reports, 27,* 1–43.

Holland, J., Ramazanoglu, J. G., Scott, S., Sharpe, S., & Thomson, R. (1991). Between embarrassment and trust: Young women and the diversity of condom use. In P. Appleton, P. Davies, & G. Hurt (Eds.), *AIDS: Responses emergency and care* (pp. 127–148). London: Routledge.

Holmes, S., & Holmes, R. (2002). *Sex crimes: Patterns and behaviors* (2nd ed.). Thousand Oaks, CA: Sage Publications.

Holtzman, C. G. (1994). Multicultural perspectives on counseling victims of rape. *Journal of Social Distress and the Homeless, 3,* 87–97.

Ingram, K., Betz, N. E., Mindes, E. J., Schmitt, M. M., & Smith, N. G. (2001). Unsupportive responses from others concerning a stressful life event: Development of the unsupportive social interactions inventory. *Journal of Social and Clinical Psychology, 20,* 173–207.

Janoff-Bulman, R. (1992). *Shattered assumption: Towards a new psychology of trauma.* New York: Free Press.

Kahn, A. S., Mathie, V. A., & Torgler, C. (1994). Rape scripts and rape acknowledgement. *Psychology of Women Quarterly, 18,* 53–66.

Kleim, B., & Ehlers, A. (2009). Evidence for a curvilinear relationship between post-traumatic growth and posttrauma depression and PTSD in assault survivors. *Journal of Traumatic Stress, 22,* 45–52.

Koss, M. P. (1985). The hidden rape victim: Personality, attitudinal, and situational characteristics. *Psychology of Women Quarterly, 9,* 193–212.

Koss, M. P. (1988). Women's mental health agenda: Violence against women. *Women's Mental Health Occasional Paper Series.* Washington DC: National Institute of Mental Health.

Koss, M. P. (2000). Blame, shame, and community: Justice responses to violence against women. *American Psychologist, 55,* 1332–1343.

Koss, M. P., & Dinero, T. E. (1989). Discriminant analysis of risk factors for sexual victimization among a national sample of college women. *Journal of Consulting and Clinical Psychology, 57,* 242–250.

Koss, M. P., Dinero, T. E., Seibel, C. A., & Cox, S. L. (1988). Stranger and acquaintance rape: Are there differences in victim's experience? *Psychology of Women Quarterly, 12,* 1–24.

Koss, M. P., & Harvey, M. R. (1991). *The rape victim: Clinical and community interventions* (2nd ed.). New York: Sage.

Koss, M. P., Heise, L., & Russo, N. (1994). The global health burden of rape. *Psychology of Women Quarterly, 18,* 509–537.

Koss, M. P., Leonard, K., Beezley, D. & Oros, C. (1985). Non-stranger sexual aggression: A discriminant analysis of the psychological characteristics of undetected offenders. *Sex Roles, 12,* 981–992.

Krahe, B. (1991). Police officers' definitions of rape: A prototype study. *Journal of Community and Applied Social Psychology, 1,* 223–244.

Krahe, B., Schutze, S., Fritsche, J. & Waizenhofer, E. (2000). The prevalence of sexual aggression and victimization among homosexual men. *Journal of Sex Research, 37,* 142–150.

Lamb, S. (1996). *The trouble with blame.* Cambridge: Harvard University Press.

Lees, S. (1986). *Losing out: Sexuality and adolescent girls.* Dover, NH: Hutchinson Publishing.

Lefley, H. P., Scott, C. S., Llabre, M., & Hicks, D. (1993). Cultural beliefs about rape and victims' response in three ethnic groups. *American Journal of Orthopsychiatry, 63,* 623–632.

Lerner, M. J. (1980). *Belief in a just world.* New York: Plenum.

Lewin, M. (1985). Unwanted intercourse: The difficulty of saying no. *Psychology of Women Quarterly, 9,* 184–192.

Linley, P. A., & Joseph, S. (2004). Positive change following trauma and adversity: A review. *Journal of Traumatic Stress, 17,* 11–21.

Littleton, H., & Axsom, D. (2003). Rape and seduction scripts of university students: Implications for rape attributions and unacknowledged rape. *Sex Roles, 49,* 465–475.

Littleton, H., Horsley, A., John, S., & Nelson, D. V. (2007). Trauma coping strategies and psychological distress: A meta-analysis. *Journal of Traumatic Stress, 20,* 977–988.

Logan, T. K., Evans, L., Stevenson, E., & Jordan, C. (2005). Barriers to services for rural and urban rape survivors. *Journal of Interpersonal Violence, 20,* 591–616.

Lonsway, K. (1996). Preventing acquaintance rape through education: What do we know? *Psychology of Women Quarterly, 20,* 229–265.

Lott, B. (1994). *Women's lives: Themes and variations in gender learning.* Pacific Grove, CA: Brooks/Cole.

Malamuth, N. M. (1984). Aggression against women: Cultural and individual causes. In N. M. Malamuth & E. Donerstein (Eds.), *Pornography and sexual aggression* (pp. 19–52). Orlando, FL: Academic.

Malamuth, N. M., & Check, J. V. P. (1985). The effects of aggressive pornography on beliefs in rape myths: Individual differences. *Journal of Research in Personality, 19,* 299–320.

McCauley, J. L., Ruggeiro, K. J., Resnick, H. S., & Kilpatrick, D. G. (2010). Incapacitated, forcible, and drug/alcohol-facilitated rape in relation to binge drinking, marijuana use, and illicit drug use: A national survey. *Journal of Traumatic Stress, 23,* 132–140.

McHugh, M. C., Watson, B., & Sullivan, H. (2009, August). Slut! Qualitative studies of the sexual double standard. Presented in panel at Research with Disadvantaged Women—Qualitative Methods as a Generative Choice (Mary Gergen, Chair), American Psychological Association, Toronto.

Mori, L., Bernat, J. A., Glenn, P. A., Selle, L. L., & Zarate, M. G. (1995). Attitudes towards rape: Gender and ethnic differences across Asian and Caucasian college students. *Sex Roles, 32,* 457–467.

Muehlenhard, C. (1988). 'Nice women' don't say yes and 'real men' don't say no: How miscommunication and the double standard can cause sexual problems. *Women & Therapy, 7,* 95–108.

Norris, F., & Kaniasty, K. (1992). A longitudinal study of the effects of various crime prevention programs on criminal victimization, fear of crime, and psychological distress. *American Journal of Community Psychology, 20,* 625–648.

Paludi, M. A. (Ed.). (1999). *The psychology of sexual victimization.* Westport, CT: Greenwood.

Park, C. L., & Helgeson, V. S. (2006). Growth following highly stressful life events: Current status and future directions. *Journal of Consulting and Clinical Psychology, 74,* 791–796.

Rozee, P. D. (2000). Sexual victimization: Harassment and rape. In M. Biaggio & M. Hersen (Eds.), *Issues in psychology of women* (pp. 93–113). New York: Kluwer.

Rozee, P. D. (2003). Women's fear of rape: Causes, consequences and coping. In J. Chrisler, C. Golden, & P. Rozee (Eds.), *Lectures in the psychology of women* (3rd ed., pp. 332–355). New York: McGraw-Hill.

Rozee, P., & Koss, M. P. (2001). Rape: A century of resistance. *Psychology of Women Quarterly, 25,* 295–311.

Rozee, P., & Van Boemel, G. (1995). The psychological effects of war trauma and abuse among older refugee women. *Women and Therapy, 8,* 23–50.

Russell, D. (1982). *Rape in marriage.* New York: Macmillan.

Sanday, P. (1981). The socio-cultural context of rape: A cross-cultural study. *Journal of Social Issues, 37,* 5–27.

Scully, D., & Marolla, J. (1998). "Riding the bull at Gilley's": Convicted rapists describe the rewards of rape. In M. E. Oden & J. Clay-Warner (Eds.), *Confronting rape and sexual assault* (pp. 109–128). Wilmington, DE: Scholarly Resources.

Simon, W., & Gagnon, J. (1984). Sexual scripts. *Society, 22,* 52–60.
Simon, W., & Gagnon, J. (1986). Sexual scripts: Permanence and change. *Archives of Sexual Behavior, 15,* 97–120.
Taylor, S. E., & Armor, D. A. (1996). Positive illusions and coping with adversity. *Journal of Personality, 64,* 873–898.
Tiefer, L. (1995). *Sex is not a natural act.* New York: Westview.
Tjaden, P., & Thoennes, N. (1998). Prevalence, incidence, and consequences of violence against women: Findings from the National Violence Survey (No. NCJ 172837). Washington, DC: U.S. Department of Justice, National Institute of Justice.
Tyra, P. A. (1993). Older women: Victims of rape. *Journal of Gerontological Nursing, 19,* 7–12.
Ulman, S. E. (2010). *Talking about sexual assault: Society's response to survivors.* Washington, DC: American Psychological Association.
Vishnevsky, T., Cann, A., Calhoun, L. G., Tedeschi, R. G., & Demakis, G. J. (2010). Gender differences in self-reported post-traumatic growth: A meta-analysis. *Psychology of Women Quarterly, 34,* 110–120.
Wyatt, G. E. (1992). The sociocultural context of African American and White American women's rape. *Journal of Social Issues, 48,* 77–91.
Yalom, I. D., & Liberman, M. A. (1991). Bereavement and heightened existential awareness. *Psychiatry, 54,* 334–345.

Chapter 2

Sexual Abuse of Girls and the Lasting Effects

Wesley S. Parks, Paula K. Lundberg-Love, and Desiree L. Glaze

INTRODUCTION

Childhood sexual abuse, once a taboo subject discussed only behind closed doors, has made its way into mainstream consciousness. As more and more women bravely come forward, telling their stories, sharing their horrors, and seeking treatment to improve their lives, our collective knowledge of the lasting effects of this heinous crime have solidified. The literature on child sexual abuse (CSA) is replete with clinical observations and lists of symptoms and disorders thought to be associated with a history of abuse. It would be all too easy to conceptualize the adult victims of CSA in such clinical terms, but that would be shortsighted and would not encourage insight into the complexities of the impact of sexual abuse. This chapter focuses on accepting the pandemic that is childhood sexual abuse and considers the theoretical framework for how sexual abuse impacts survivors and understanding the lasting effects of childhood sexual abuse on adult women survivors.

DEFINING THE PROBLEM

Almost any approach to a scientific understanding of phenomena begins with the most basic step of defining the problem. The federal definition of child abuse was outlined in the Federal Child Abuse and Prevention and Treatment Act (CAPTA), as amended by the Keeping Children and Families Safe Act of 2003. Sexual abuse is defined by CAPTA as "the employment, use, persuasion, inducement, enticement, or coercion of any child to engage in, or assist any other person to engage in, any sexually explicit conduct or simulation of such conduct for the purpose of producing a visual depiction of such conduct; or the rape, and in cases of caretaker or inter-familial relationships, statutory rape, molestation, prostitution, or other form of sexual exploitation of children, or incest with children" (United States Department of Health and Human Services, 2008, p. 1). The federal definition of sexual abuse includes activities by a parent or caregiver such as fondling a child's genitals, penetration, incest, rape, sodomy, indecent exposure, and exploitation through prostitution or the production of pornographic materials. It was further noted that each state provides its own definitions of child abuse and neglect based on the federally mandated minimum standard set forth in CAPTA. Walker, Carey, Mohr, Stein, & Seddat (2004) cited a prior definition set forth by the federal government in 1981 that also included "an act by another minor when that person is either significantly older than the victim (often defined as more than 5 years) or when the perpetrator is in a position of power or control over the child." Interestingly, the age stipulation is no longer included in the federal definition of CSA, although many states have their own statutes addressing this point.

What is clear from the federally standardized definition is an obvious lack of specificity for such terms as "penetration," "sodomy," and "exposure." This is just the beginning of the epidemiological problem of researching CSA. Browne and Finkelhor (1986), in a review of more than 25 published studies of the effects of CSA, noted a wide variation in the definitions of CSA. This variability included not only a lack of consistency in how sexual behavior was defined but also variability in factors such as inclusion of noncontact events, the ages of the victim and perpetrator, whether the event was wanted or unwanted, and even whether or not the perpetrator was a family member. A cursory review of some of these studies, which are not cited in this chapter because their information is not integrated into this chapter aside from this one notation, also suggest a tendency to weigh penetrative acts more heavily than nonpenetrative acts, possibly implying that sexual assaults that did not include actual oral, vaginal, or anal penetration may not have been as significant as penetrative abuse. That is, unless the act involves contact by an older perpetrator, there is a risk that it will be viewed as less serious or less traumatic and is thereby excluded from data sets. Lemeiux and Byers (2008) quite correctly stated that research in this area has been plagued by various methodological problems, including operational definitions. Trying to agree on a concrete operational definition of CSA is all but impossible, as some researchers reject a database that does not include contact abuse or that focuses on same-age peers. The obvious problem with this lack of clarity is that we are at risk of overlooking entire subsets of data because they do not conform to the previously established and what could be considered a male-centric conceptualization of CSA. While there can be no doubt that the level of physical intrusiveness has an impact on a female's sexual identity and well-being, the notion that less intrusive experiences cannot be equally traumatic is disturbing.

PREVALENCE OF CSA

Without a clear-cut definition of CSA, it is all but impossible to find agreed-upon published prevalence rates for CSA. Cortina and Kubiak (2006) cited previous conservative estimates that one in four American women experiences sexual violence at some point in her lifetime, including forced rape. Many women experience multiple forms of sexual violence throughout adulthood, and childhood sexual abuse increases the risk of future sexual violence in adolescents and adults (Cortina and Kubiak, 2006). In a longitudinal study published in 2000, Humphrey and White (2000) found that 36% of college women reported some type of childhood sexual abuse, and nearly 50% reported at least one victimization experience in high school. In a subset study by McMullin, Wirth, and White (2007) of Humphrey and White's original data, 19% of participants reported that across their life spans the most severe form of sexual victimization experienced was rape, 13.3% reported coerced sexual contact, 15.8% reported attempted rape, and 51.9% reported unwanted sexual contact (McMullin et al., 2007).

Wyatt and Peters (1986) reviewed four then well-cited studies of prevalence rates of CSA. They noted that the four studies used different definitions of CSA when determining prevalence rates. When they recomputed the rates using the most stringent definition of the four studies, the result lowered the prevalence rate by at least 8%. Roosa, Reyes, Reinholtz, and Angelini (1998) used eight newly created measures of sexual abuse and found incidence rates ranging from 18% to 59%, depending on the measure used. In general, the more types of CSA included in a measure, the higher the number of women who reported CSA. When boyfriends and spouses were eliminated as perpetrators, the rate dropped by 50%. Without a clear-cut definition, various interviewers, law enforcement officials, legal officials, and mental health professions are apt to miscategorize certain instances of abuse. Hence, the resulting prevalence rates may not be accurate.

The most recent data from the United States Department of Health and Human Services (2010) is a report titled *Child Maltreatment 2010,* which is a yearly update of the statistics of all reported and investigated instances of child abuse and neglect in all 50 states. In 2008 there were 69,184 reported instances of CSA. This represents 9.1% of the total reported abuse and neglect cases for that year's data set. When compared to the U.S. Census Bureau population estimates from that same time period (United States Census Bureau, 2008), the reported and investigated abuse represented less than 1% of the U.S. population of children and adolescents. It should be noted that these data included only cases that were reported and investigated by state agencies and did not include any self-reports that were not investigated.

The number of sexual abuse cases substantiated by state agencies dropped by 40% from 1992 to 2000 (Finkelhor and Jones, 2004). Finkelhor, undeniably a leader in the research of CSA, found such a sharp decline to be all but impossible to understand. Cited were numerous plausible explanations, including better reporting statistics, overall decline in crimes against children, the effectiveness of prevention programs, and the decline in self-reported yet unsubstantiated outcries. In the end, the authors concluded that further study was needed to determine the true prevalence rates of these crimes and understand what problems, social or legal, might have contributed to the decline and the extent to which that may have occurred. Regardless of the possible reasons, it was believed that there was a genuine decline in the incidence of substantiated cases of CSA. The likely consequence, at least suggested by Finkelhor and Jones, would include less focus on CSA in the future. If there is less of a focus on the abuse itself, it stands to reason that there would also be the potential for less focus on the effects of the abuse.

All of this fails to address the number of unreported cases of CSA. It is important to keep in mind that published literature about CSA requires data input from victims who agree to participate. In random sampling models where a large number of people are contacted and given the opportunity to participate, these initial contacts are focused on a set population based on what has already been reported, such as targeting those who are in survivors groups, or are based on contacting a large demographic, such as first-year college students, and hoping for a high hit rate. These methods of recruitment rely on women coming forward themselves or admitting to abuse when given an opportunity to do so. This does not include women who are prone to denying any form of abuse, for whatever reason, and thus these data may never paint an accurate picture in terms of the actual prevalence of CSA or its lasting effects.

TRAUMAGENIC MODEL

Understanding the effects of any type of abuse, including CSA, requires a conceptual framework. The most widely cited model in the articles reviewed for this chapter (Lemieux and Byers, 2008; Liem, O'Toole & James, 1992; Feerick and Snow, 2005; Horowitz, Widom, McLaughlin, & White, 2001; Gibson & Leitenberg, 2001; Arata, 2002; Kendall-Tackett, Williams, and Finkelhor, 1993) was the traumagenic dynamics model first proposed by Finkelhor and Browne (1985).

The following overview of the model is taken directly from Finkelhor and Browne's (1985) conceptualization and is important to understand when considering the immediate and lasting effects of CSA. The traumagenic model can be thought of as four discrete factors: traumatic sexualization, betrayal, powerlessness, and stigmatization. As the authors noted, these dynamics are not unique to CSA and can be applied to any manner of trauma. Nevertheless, this seems to be the best model for understanding how children's eventual self-concept, affective responses to the world, and psychological and psychiatric well-being can be impacted by sexual abuse. Understanding the underpinnings of the lasting effects rather than just rattling off a list of possible symptoms and outcomes can assist in shaping more effective treatments and may well serve the public policy debates that focus on prevention.

TRAUMATIC SEXUALIZATION

Traumatic sexualization is itself a two-part process for the development of the traumatic component. The first prong begins with the sexualization of the child, which occurs when a child engages in sexual behavior that is developmentally inappropriate. This can include exchanged sex for affection, attention, basic needs (food, clothing), gifts, etc. It can also include the fetishizing of a child or her anatomy. The second part of the traumatic prong can occur with the physical act of the abuse, when the child has misconceptions about the behavior or the wrongfulness of what has previously occurred, or through frightening events and memories that become associated with the sexual activity. Finkelhor and Browne note that children who have been traumatically sexualized often engage in inappropriate sexual behavior, have misconceptions about sexual self-concepts, and attach unusual emotional associations with sex.

Betrayal

Betrayal, simply put, occurs when a child realizes that a person she was dependent on or who had influence over her has caused her harm. The betrayal can come in the form of feeling betrayed by the actual perpetrator or by those who did not participate but are viewed at sources of protection, such as parents who were not able to stop the abuse of which they may have been unaware and those who knew of the abuse but did nothing to stop it. After the abuse, betrayal can continue when attitudes toward the victim change after the disclosure.

Powerlessness

Powerlessness is alternatively called disempowerment (Finkelhor and Browne, 1985). The authors noted that there are many potential aspects of the experience that can lead to feelings of powerlessness, not the least of which is the violation of the child's body. Disempowerment can also develop when manipulation or coercion is employed, when the abuse occurs more than once, when a child is unable to make an outcry or is not believed when making an outcry, and especially when the perpetrator is in some position of authority over the child, such as a trusted family friend, teacher, minister, etc. The powerlessness facet of this model comprises mechanisms similar to post-traumatic stress disorder (PTSD), such as an intense fear of death or uncontrollable injury. There is also the repeated frustration of not being able to stop the event or escape from the situation (Kendall-Tackett, Williams, and Finkelhor, 1993). However, when children are able to bring the abuse to an end, they can regain some sense of empowerment.

Stigmatization

The final dynamic is stigmatization which includes shame, guilt and badness that are communicated to children that eventually become part of their self-concept and self-image (Finkelhor and Browne, 1985). The negative connotations can be communicated directly or indirectly. They are reinforced by the attitudes that the child infers or hears, which adds to her own knowledge that the event was in fact a taboo or forbidden experience. When considering children's social cognition, it is important to note that they are active processors of social information. They look to others for social cues and are constantly drawing inferences and formulating explanations for what they observe (Siegler, DeLoache, and Eisenberg, 2003). Hence, stigmatization can be the most troublesome of the four dynamics because it involves the internalization of others' reactions to the abuse in addition to the feelings of the child.

IMPACT OF ABUSE IN TRAUMAGENIC MODEL

Any review of the literature on CSA culminates in a list of symptoms, disorders, and possible outcomes. This certainly was the case in reviewing the materials for this chapter and is to be expected given that mental health symptoms and diagnoses are made based on a categorical model as outlined in the *Diagnostic and Statistical Manual of Mental Disorders,* 4th ed. (*DSM-IV-TR*). Undoubtedly, a list of symptoms is necessary to diagnose a disorder and structure a treatment plan. In fact, the Task Force for *DSM-IV* noted that the *DSM* is structured categorically rather than dimensionally in an effort to organize and transmit diagnostic and treatment information. However, the *DSM-IV-TR* also notes the limitations of such a model, especially given the variability of clinical presentation (American Psychiatric Association, 2000). The benefit of the traumagenic model in understanding the lasting effects of CSA is that it does not rely on a categorical list of symptoms such as would be needed to diagnose PTSD. Rather, the traumagenic model incorporates the underlying causes of the symptoms and can be beneficial in making clinical assessments of the possible effects of CSA (Finkelhor and Browne, 1985). When looking at the lasting effects of CSA, including the manifestation of past and present symptoms, it is important to consider the totality of the experience that led to the symptoms rather than considering just the abusive act itself. Feinauer, Middleton, and Hilton (2003) wrote that current and past research has shown a correlation between the severity of abuse and the degree of psychological trauma. Keeping that framework in the forefront of our minds will be important in order for understanding how the lasting effects of CSA develop and also for understanding their potency for psychological devastation.

Lasting Effects of CSA

In reviewing the National Comorbidity Study, Mulder et al. (1998) found that when statistical methods were utilized to control for other childhood adversities, there were significant correlations between CSA and 14 mood, anxiety, and substance abuse disorders in women. In the same study in a subsample reporting no other adversities, there were higher rates of depression and substance abuse with victims of CSA. As would be expected, that same study also revealed that rape, personal association with the perpetrator, and repeated incidents of CSA were associated with higher incidents of diagnosable disorders. Kendler et al. (2000) found that any CSA, regardless of background or other contributing factors, was associated with major depressive disorder, generalized anxiety disorder, panic disorder, and substance abuse. Although there are confounds with CSA and other risk factors, there is a commonality between diagnosable disorders and CSA. This implies that regardless of other factors, CSA alone can contribute to diagnosable disorders, and likely the clinically significant symptoms are intensified when confounds are present.

Many of the lasting effects of CSA may stem from short-term or immediate clinical concerns that were never resolved. For example, consider the development of PTSD. What happens when a diagnosis is made but no treatment is given or treatment is ineffective? As with any disorder, the symptoms may continue to some degree. It stands to reason, then, that if a child has PTSD from sexual abuse, it could carry over into adulthood as a lasting effect of CSA. The same is likely true for other disorders as well (anxiety disorder, mood disorders, etc.). Given that the *DSM-IV-TR,* the current method for diagnosis of mental health disorders, separated disorders categorically, it is helpful to consider the lasting effects of CSA categorically as well where applicable, such as specific disorder sets. However, some of the most severe lasting effects, such as sexual identity concerns and revictimization, are not associated with specific disorder sets and are discussed in terms of global effects.

Anxiety Disorders

Inarguably the most common lasting effect associated with CSA is anxiety disorders and specifically PTSD. Most of the research in PTSD has focused on adults, but more studies have been added in the past 20 years that examine childhood development of PTSD. Dubner and Motta (1999), in their review of the literature in 1999, found then-recent studies to show PTSD in sexually abused children from rates as low as 0% to as high as 90%. They noted that the disparity likely stemmed from numerous factors, including the measures used, the demographic variability, accuracy of self-reporting, classification of abuse, etc., some of the same variables that contribute to the lack of accurate reporting of CSA in general. In their study of sexually abused foster care children, Dubner and Motta (1999) found that 60% of their sample met the diagnostic criteria for PTSD. It should be noted that their sample included boys and girls. In another study by McLeer, Deblinger, Atkins, Foa, and Ralphe (1988) that included four times as many sexually abused girls as it did boys, the authors found that 48% met the criteria for PTSD. Finkelhor and Browne (1985) estimated that between 46% and 66% of children who were sexually abused exhibited significant psychological impairment, including anxiety symptoms.

In contrast, there are those who suggest that perhaps there are not enough criteria met for a diagnosis of PTSD in children or that the criteria cannot be uniformly applied to all instances of sexual abuse. In theory, PTSD arises from experiences that are overwhelming, sudden, and dangerous. According to Kendall-Tackett et al. (1993), many cases of sexual abuse lack these components, and therefore a diagnosis of PTSD would not be appropriate. In an analysis by McNally (1993) of six studies that applied PTSD criteria to CSA, only two of the four studies reported any cases of PTSD. Cortina and Kubiak (2006) reviewed one of the most widely cited epidemiological studies of gender differences in PTSD. They believed that the lack of specificity in the screening process in addition to broad categorical ranges led to the faulty conclusion set forth by earlier research that there was an inherent feminine vulnerability to PTSD-like symptoms and that those studies therefore underestimated the genuine prevalence of PTSD (Cortina and Kubiak, 2006) in girls. Instead, the studies attributed symptoms to other more histrionic-like behavior. Putnam (2009) reviewed several studies and put forth a list of possible indicators of PTSD: fearfulness, anxiety states, sleep disturbances, nightmares, psychosomatic complaints, phobic avoidance of males if the perpetrator was male, reliving the event, and avoiding activities reminiscent of the event. What is clear, even in studies that question the appropriateness of PTSD diagnosis in children, is that an argument can be made that these children nonetheless experience PTSD symptoms even if not to a diagnostically specific level. One question that this evokes reinforces the importance of strong data for both CSA events and resulting symptoms: Is the lack of appropriate classification of traumatic events and subsequent symptoms altering the true prevalence rates for diagnoses of PTSD?

Koverola and Foy (1993) noted that one controversy surrounding PTSD diagnoses in child victims of sexual abuse is that children manifest symptoms differently from adults and argue that children are less likely to have dissociative flashbacks and are more likely to experience nightmares. With respect to nightmares, Terr (1989) has argued in her presentation to the DSM-IV Work Group on PTSD that there are two distinct types. Type I nightmares are graphic representations of a single original traumatic event. These typically appear soon after the abuse and decrease over time. Type II nightmares are symbolic representations of the traumatic event and may include denial, dissociation, and numbing. These nightmares may exceed Type I nightmares and may continue well into adulthood.

Feerick and Snow (2005) examined how the characteristics of sexual abuse, rather than simply categorizing respondents as abused or nonabused, were related to lasting effects of CSA after childhood and adolescence. In their survey of 313 undergraduate women, 31% reported some form of childhood sexual abuse.

A post hoc analysis of the reported symptoms indicated that women who had experienced either attempted or completed intercourse reported more PTSD symptoms than nonabused women. Not surprisingly, Feerick and Snow found that the symptoms of PTSD increased as the severity of the abuse increased. It was lowest in women with no abuse, higher in women who had experienced exposure (flashing), higher still in those who had been fondled and touched, and highest when any type of penetration had occurred. The age of the individual at the time of abuse also was statistically significant. The younger a victim was when she was abused, the fewer numbers of PTSD symptoms were obtained, but higher numbers of symptoms of avoidance and distress were reported. It was noted that the age of onset of abuse and the symptoms of avoidance and distress were similar to those obtained in prior research studies. However, Feerick and Snow indicated that their results contraindicated prior research showing a correlation with greater PTSD symptoms in adulthood when the victimization occurred at a younger age. They suggested several possibilities for these discrepancies, including the generally accepted notion that PTSD symptoms decline over time, with the most severe symptoms being experienced immediately after the event. Thus, a college-age woman in their study who suffered abuse at age 5 versus age 15 might have had longer to develop coping skills to offset PTSD symptoms. Also, higher reports of distress may stem from the higher rates of feeling pressured to participate during the abuse, as this is an intrapersonal anxiety response, and PTSD is a response to external stimuli. Hence, avoidance and distress may still be high in those reporting earlier onset of abuse because interpersonal identities are more formative in younger years and thus are susceptible to long-term damage.

After the release of the National Comorbidity Survey (NCS) in 2001, many researchers began analyzing data for the presence of psychological disorders as a function of numerous variables, including CSA. Molnar, Buka, and Kessler (2001) found that of the women who reported a history of CSA, 39.1% met the criteria for PTSD, as compared to 5.7% who did not report a history of CSA. In comparison with all other domains tapped by the NCS diagnostic criteria, PTSD was the second-highest diagnosis met by women reporting CSA. Only depression was more prevalent (39.3%). While 78% of the women met criteria for one or more disorders, the number who still met PTSD criteria years after their abuse experiences was remarkable. One explanation may be the coping strategies utilized by these women. Gibson and Leitenberg (2001) found that those who used disengagement (avoidance, wishful thinking, social withdrawal, self-criticism, etc.) as a coping style maintained PTSD and continued to experience general psychological distress. Alternatively, even without employing disengagement strategies, a lack of appropriate therapeutic interventions and a paucity of engagement behaviors serve to prolong the course of the disorder. Walsh, Blaustein, Knight, Spinazzola, and van der Kolk (2007) found that women who engaged in cognitive coping strategies were more emotionally adjusted than women who used disengagement strategies. Not surprising to mental health professionals, adult female survivors with PTSD who sought and completed treatment showed a reduction in PTSD symptoms. There are numerous studies to support the efficacy of treatment (e.g., Rowan and Foy, 2003; Elklit, 2009; Cohen, 2008; Himelein and McElrath, 1996; and McDonagh et al. 2005).

Affective Disorders

Based on Molnar, Buka, and Kessler's (2001) review of the NCS, there was a significant correlation between affective disorders and women with a history of CSA. Of the respondents, 39.3% met the criteria for depression, 15.7% met the criteria for dysthymia, and 1.4% met the criteria for mania. Prior to Molnar, Buka, and Kessler's study, Browne and Finkelhor (1986) conducted a thorough review of the literature regarding the impact of CSA. They highlighted two community-based studies that showed higher rates of depression in women who suffered CSA as compared to nonabused women and also discussed four other clinical studies that showed at least moderate, if not significant, elevations in depression among female survivors of CSA. Hyun, Freedman, and Dunner (2000) found higher rates of bipolar and unipolar disorder in both men and women with histories of CSA. However, such numbers were higher in women than in men. As this study included physical abuse as a variable, it is noteworthy that bipolar and unipolar disorders were higher for victims of sexual abuse than for victims of physical abuse, suggesting that sexual abuse may be more traumatic than physical abuse. There has been some debate regarding whether or not age at the time of abuse or severity of abuse affected the correlations. Walker et al. (2004) found inconsistencies in correlations between the age of abuse and the severity of symptoms, noting that some studies showed that younger ages of abuse contributed to greater levels of severe symptomatology, while other studies showed no such correlation. Whatever the reality is and regardless of the age of the onset of abuse or the level of the severity of abuse, mood symptoms are a prominent lasting effect in women.

Substance Abuse

Clay, Olsheski, and Clay (2000) reviewed research that suggested contributory factors in the development of alcohol-use disorders in women who were sexually abused as children. The authors identified several correlates between CSA and substance abuse. Age at the time of abuse was correlated with higher prevalence rates of alcohol-use disorder (AUD). The limited number of studies that have examined the relationship between the age of the victim at the time of the sexual abuse and the likelihood of developing alcohol-use disorder later in life have generally suggested that the younger the victim is at the time of the abuse, the less likely she is to later develop an AUD. Clay et al. suggested that younger victims had less memory for the events or had developed other coping methods by the time they first tried alcohol. The Jarvis study as well as two others cited in this review suggested a higher incidence of AUD when the abuse occurred at age 10 or later.

With respect to the duration and severity of abuse, the limited research found by Clay et al. (2000) suggests that the more severe the abuse (e.g., penetrative versus unwanted kissing) and the longer the abuse occurred, the more likely is the development of AUD in adulthood. CSA perpetrated by males has been linked to the development of AUD in adult females regardless of the known identity (father figure versus stranger).

Studies examining self-esteem did not find significant differences between those with and without AUD. Clay et al. (2000) attribute this to prior findings that CSA survivors generally have lower self-esteem anyway, regardless of later psychopathology. Those with an external locus of control (LOC), individuals who believe that their environment, powerful others, fate, or even chance determine the events in their lives, are more likely to abuse alcohol, which may be to overcome stigma and powerlessness. Some studies showed higher rates of AUD among survivors of multiple CSA encounters. Those who sought help after disclosing incest were less likely to develop AUD. This study did note that CSA and AUD are often diagnosed by different professionals with different training. Diagnostic cross-training may increase the specificity of diagnoses. For example, those treating AUD might uncover more CSA if trained to gather complete trauma histories.

Kendler et al.'s (2000) epidemiological study of CSA and adult psychiatric disorders and substance abuse disorders in female twins indicated significant correlations between CSA and alcohol dependence and drug dependence, with odds ratios being as high as 5.7. The odds ratios increased as the dimension of the severity of abuse increased (nongenital, genital, intercourse). The NCS results (Molnar et al., 2001) indicated that for women with histories of CSA, 33.9% met the criteria for alcohol problems, 15.6% met the criteria for alcohol dependence, 7.4% met the criteria for severe alcohol dependence, 27.6% met the criteria for drug problems, 14.1% met the criteria for drug dependence, and 9.8% met the criteria for severe drug dependence. Davidson and van der Kolk (2007) found that patients with PTSD-related problems have high rates of self-medication, including the use of alcohol or illicit substances. Given the overlap between PTSD in adult survivors of CSA and the prevalence rates of substance use in this population, it is important for clinicians to recall that these women frequently may use alcohol or other substances as a coping mechanism.

Personality Factors

Personality traits are enduring patterns of thinking about and relating to one's environment that are exhibited in a wide range of interpersonal and social frameworks. Personality traits are characterological and therefore tend to remain stable over time. Perhaps the most distinct personality disorder associated with CSA is borderline personality disorder (BPD). BPD is at its core instability in interpersonal relationships, self-image, affectivity, and behaviors. Individuals with BPD make frantic efforts to avoid abandonment, real or imagined. Their interpersonal relations are intense and are characterized by alternating from extremes of idealization to devaluation. There tends to be an unstable self-image. Recurrent suicidal, parasuicidal, or self-harm behaviors are common. Affective instability from mood lability is prominent. An inability to control anger, often intense and inappropriate anger, is common. Feelings of emptiness are prominent. In addition, some individuals with BPD may experience paranoid ideation or, rarely, dissociative symptoms.

Traumatic sexualization, as a factor in the traumagenic model, often results in confusion about the role of sex in relationships (Finkelhor and Browne, 1985). If the child traded sex for affection over time, this pattern of gaining affection may become the baseline and could result in idealizing the abuser when "love" is shown and devaluing the abuser after the event. When considering the powerlessness component of the traumagenic model, the expectation of being revictimized may lead to affective instability and suicidal gestures (Finkelhor and Browne, 1985).

In Browne and Finkelhor's (1985) study on the impact of child abuse, the emotional reactions and self-perceptions in the long-term effects of CSA survivors were emphasized. While the authors did not specifically identify any particular personality disorder, their description of what was reported at community clinics and in prior research studies suggests the possibility of an association of CSA and BPD. They reported one particular community sample wherein 51% of abused victims reported a history of suicide attempts, 64% reported feelings of isolation, and 54% reported anxiety or tension. Taken at face value, these findings do not necessarily support the notion of a personality disorder, but those symptoms can be associated with BPD or other personality disorders. In considering the overlap between BPD and PTSD, Landecker (1992) noted that neither diagnosis adequately addressed the symptoms of most people with CSA histories. PTSD does not take into account the characterological dysfunction in response to severe abuse experiences, and BPD attributes symptoms solely to such dysfunction in lieu of recognizing the adaptive component afforded by a PTSD diagnosis. In short, sometimes there is leeway for the clinician to offer one diagnosis over another, which may be incorrect, or to preclude the possibility of both diagnoses.

Feinauer, Callahan, and Hilton (1996) cited several previous studies that established a correlation between childhood sexual abuse and difficulty forming or maintaining interpersonal relationships. They noted that interpersonal difficulties are generally presented anecdotally rather than empirically and thus are inferential in nature. Their study, which included an empirical measure of relationship satisfaction, found that as intimate relationships became less well adjusted, depression increased. The study supported previously published data that healthy relationships can be useful in alleviating the symptoms of depression in CSA survivors and also found that level of depression increased with the severity of the abuse, as did the interpersonal difficulties. Thus, the more severe the abuse, the greater the severity of the adult depression and the greater the difficulty in maintaining intimate relationships. Yet when these relationships are maintained, they can be useful in alleviating the symptoms of depression.

In a Danish study of women with CSA, Kristensen and Lau (2007) reference a meta-analysis that reviewed six population studies and found that female survivors of CSA were less likely than nonvictims to be married and had smaller social networks. Kristensen and Lau (2007) in their own study found that CSA survivors were less likely to be in an intimate relationship, were less likely to be employed, and were less well educated and less well-off financially than a random sample of Danish women. As could be expected, Kristensen and Lau also found a high rate of psychiatric symptoms (such as depression) that was consistent with numerous other published studies. One limitation of their study was the high percentage of CSA victims who experienced incest. Interestingly, a large percentage of their study (20%) declined group therapy for incest, and another 66% of those who agreed to treatment never showed up for therapy. Kristensen and Lau also noted that two-thirds of the women in their study previously had undergone some form of treatment. The authors felt that while their results were not generalizable to all Danish women who suffered CSA, they believed that the results did support the need for social and psychiatric intervention so that women could achieve greater levels of social functioning and occupational status.

Somaticism

Almost every study reviewed that discussed the lasting effects of CSA mentions the issue of somatic complaints, such as sleep disorders and eating disorders (e.g., Molnar et al., 2001; Browne and Finkelhor, 1985; Kendall-Tackett et al., 1993; Nelson, 2002). In fact, when considering possible outcomes of CSA, the list almost always includes somatic complaints of some form even if casually related to other disorders (e.g., sleep difficulties as related to depression.)

Nelson (2002) put forth an interesting argument that some physical complaints of women stem from CSA directly or indirectly related to the sexual acts. In her study, Nelson asked four community-based projects working with female survivors of CSA to share their most reported physical complaints. All four reported gynecological problems; respiratory problems; intestinal disorders (mostly irritable bowel syndrome); back pain; migraines; hip and joint pain; chronic pelvic pain; muscle stiffness and weakness in the jaw, neck, and shoulders; dental neglect due to dental phobia; chronic fatigue; and obesity and eating disorders. When considering the implications for why this population reported such a high number of physical complaints and why there appeared to be such overlap between physical and psychiatric symptoms in CSA survivors, Nelson considered the usual theories, including that having a physical disorder such as arthritis could lead to depression or that having a psychiatric condition such as obsessive-compulsive disorder could lead to a bowel disorder. But she put forth an interesting third possibility: that CSA could give rise to both the physical disorders and the psychiatric problems. This rationale could explain why women who suffered oral penetration later report muscle tension as adults, as their necks and shoulders were yanked around and bent backwards for oral abuse. Another example provided was the consideration of paradoxical vocal cord dysfunction in children as a marker for oral sexual abuse when no other medically observable reason can be determined, as this condition is caused by the vocal cords closing when breathing in or in response to an attack on the airway. While paradoxical vocal cord dysfunction is usually considered psychosomatic in children when asthma is not present, it may be that this is an indicator of sexual trauma. She readily admits that more research is needed in this area. However, it is an interesting hypothesis and one that many treating clinicians have considered over the years (Lundberg-Love, 1990, 1999).

Revictimization

One of the most robust findings in the research on CSA is that women who were sexually victimized in childhood are at greater risk for being victimized at other times during their life span (Lundberg-Love, 1990, 1999). Lemeiux and Byers (2008) found that 54% of women in their survey who experienced CSA with attempted or completed penetration (vaginal, oral, or anal) between the ages of 13 and 16 years were significantly more likely to report being victimized during adulthood than those who had been fondled only. The women in Gibson and Leitenberg's (2001) study with a history of CSA who suffered revictimization as adults had more feelings of powerlessness and stigmatization than women without CSA histories, thus further providing support for the traumagenic model of understanding the effects of CSA. Arata's (2002) analysis of 17 studies of the rates of revictimization found that these ranged from as low as 6% to as high as 78.6%, with the highest rates being found in the studies with the largest sample sizes.

Rich, Combs-Lane, Resnick, and Kilpatrick (2004) examined nine studies that investigated the correlation between CSA and adult sexual abuse (ASA). They found that all studies supported the phenomenon of revictimization. In each of the studies they sampled, women with CSA were significantly more likely than nonvictims to experience ASA, up to three times more likely in some studies. The authors concluded that simply having CSA increased any woman's chance for ASA. The authors did find some mediating variables that could explain this phenomenon, including higher use of illicit substances and a higher number of sexual partners in general among victims of CSA. Interestingly, these mediating variables are themselves documented lasting effects of CSA, and thus the authors' notion that they are at all mediating the risk of revictimization is questionable.

Sexual Identity Concerns

Browne and Finkelhor (1985) noted that long-term sexual functioning was an area of interest for researchers because almost all empirically based studies showed later sexual problems among CSA survivors, with the highest rates of sexual adjustment problems being present in incest survivors.

The traumagenic dynamics model proposed by Finkelhor and Browne (1985) notes that child sexual abuse shapes children's sexual attitudes and feelings in dysfunctional ways. The shaping in question can occur when children are rewarded for inappropriate sexual behavior, when they or their anatomy are fetishized, when a sexual response is evoked in the child, or when negative feelings and memories become associated with a sexual activity. Finkelhor and Browne (1985) concluded that children who endure sexual victimization are likely to experience distorted sexual cognitions, attitudes, emotions, and behaviors. It is not a stretch to assume that the greater the degree of victimization, the greater the traumatic sexualization. This is even more problematic when the event is incestuous in nature. Internalizing feelings of guilt and blame is common in survivors of CSA, as with other traumatic experiences.

Lasting effects are not well theorized, due in part to a lack of community-based research samples, and much of what has been concluded derives from learning theory, especially the classical conditioning model (Lemieux and Byers, 2008). Instrumental conditioning relies on pairing a cognitive, emotional, and/or physiological response with a stimulus. Anybody who has ever quit smoking, gained weight from emotional overeating, or seen a token economy modify a child's behavior is familiar with instrumental conditioning. At its simplest, a child raises her or his hand and a teacher calls on the child, who produces the correct answer to a question and gets praise. Every time the teacher has a question, that child's hand shoots up. It becomes automatic. The same can be true of negative consequences.

Lemieux and Byers (2008) also reviewed the limited literature of erotophilia-erotophobia and found no published research that assessed erotophobia-erotophilia among women with and without a history of CSA. In general, those with erotophobia tend to avoid sexual intimacy, engage in less autoerotic behaviors, and have more negative attitudes about their own sexuality. Finkelhor and Browne (1985) purported that early traumatic sexual experiences can alter belief systems and self-concepts, particularly with respect to sexual functioning. Hence, it is logical to conclude that women with histories of CSA might be expected to be more erotophobic.

Lemieux and Byers (2008) also reviewed several studies regarding the sexual satisfaction of adult survivors of CSA. The results were variable. Some studies reported lower sexual satisfaction in CSA survivors, while others demonstrated no such relationship. The differences could be attributed to inconsistent definitions of what constitutes sexual satisfaction. Finkelhor and Browne (1985) noted that victims of CSA often have an aversion to sex, flashbacks to the abuse experience, difficulty with arousal and orgasm, vaginismus, and negative attitudes toward their sexuality and bodies. These factors clearly can impede sexual satisfaction. Browne and Finkelhor (1986) also noted that there have been few community-based studies of sexual adjustment and sexual satisfaction. Thus, it is possible that larger community-based samples could provide richer data.

Kendall-Tackett et al. (1993) found that the frequency of sexualized behaviors in CSA victims (frequent and overt self-stimulation, inappropriate overtures, and compulsive talk, play, and fantasy with sexual content) was difficult to determine. Across six studies, sexualized behavior occurred in 35% of preschoolers and gradually tapered to 7% of older children. Authors cautioned against considering sexualized behavior as a sign of sexual abuse, as one 1989 study found that 17% of physically abused (but not sexually abused) children also exhibit sexualized behaviors. Thus, some aftermath may include sexualized behaviors but not in all cases or for all types of abuse.

CONCLUSION

To be sure, survivors of childhood sexual abuse experience myriad problems later in life. Some problems, such as PTSD, begin with the index abuse and continue into adulthood. Symptoms often begin after the event and continue to manifest into adulthood in the form of flashbacks and intrusive thoughts. Other problems, such as depressive disorders or personality disorders, can manifest in adulthood as a woman attempts to move forward with her life and relationships. Research has shown that CSA survivors can experience a host of symptoms related to affective instability, anxiety, personality traits, substance abuse, somatic concerns, revictimization, and problems with sexual identify and sexual satisfaction. When these symptoms are viewed through the lens of the traumagenic model, it is easier to understand these women as more than a list of symptoms and/or disorders. Rather, they are suffering from a traumatic childhood event that has followed them into adulthood and potentially has the power to wreak havoc on myriad aspects of their lives.

REFERENCES

American Psychiatric Association. (2000). *Diagnostic and statistical manual of mental disorders* (Revised 4th ed.). Washington, DC: American Psychiatric Association.

Arata, C. (2002). Child sexual abuse and sexual revictimization. *Clinical Psychology: Science and Practice, 9,* 135–164.

Browne, A., & Finkelhor, D. (1986). Impact of child sexual abuse: A review of the research. *Psychological Bulletin, 99,* 66–77.

Clay, K. M., Olsheski, J. A., & Clay, S. W. (2000). Alcohol use disorders in female survivors of childhood sexual abuse. *Alcoholism Treatment Quarterly, 18,* 19–29.

Cohen, J. N. (2008). Using feminist, emotion-focused and developmental approaches to enhance cognitive-behavioral therapies for post-traumatic stress disorder related to childhood sexual abuse. *Psychotherapy Theory, Research, Practice, Training, 45,* 227–246.

Cortina, L. M., & Kubiak S. P. (2006). Gender and post-traumatic stress: Sexual violence as an explanation for women's increased risk. *Journal of Abnormal Psychology, 115,* 753–759.

Davidson, J. R. T., & van der Kolk, B. A. (2007). The psychopharmacological treatment of post-traumatic stress disorder. In B. van der Kolk, A. McFarlane, & L. Weisaeth

(Eds.), *Traumatic stress: The effects of overwhelming experience on mind, body and society* (pp. 510–524). New York: Guilford.

Dubner, A. E., & Motta, R. W. (1999). Sexually and physically abused foster care children and post-traumatic stress disorder. *Journal of Consulting and Clinical Psychology, 67,* 367–373.

Elklit, A. (2009). Traumatic stress and psychological adjustment in treatment-seeking women sexually abused in childhood: A follow-up. *Scandinavian Journal of Psychology, 50,* 251–257.

Feerick, M. M., & Snow, K. L. (2005). The relationships between childhood sexual abuse, social anxiety, and symptoms of post-traumatic stress disorder in women. *Journal of Family Violence, 20,* 409–419.

Feinauer, L., Callahan, E. D., & Hilton, G. H. (1996). Positive intimate relationships decrease depression in sexually abused women. *American Journal of Family Therapy, 24,* 99–106.

Feinauer, L., Middleton, K. C., & Hilton, G. H. (2003). Existential well-being as a factor in the adjustment of adults sexually abused as children. *American Journal of Family Therapy, 31,* 201–213.

Finkelhor, D., & Browne, A. (1985). The traumatic impact of child sexual abuse: A conceptualization. *American Journal of Orthopsychiatry, 55,* 530–541.

Finkelhor, D., & Jones, L. M. (2004). Explanations for the decline in child sexual abuse cases. *Juvenile Justice Bulletin.* Washington, DC: U.S. Department of Justice.

Gibson, L., & Leitenberg, H. (2001). The impact of child sexual abuse and stigma on methods of coping with sexual assault among undergraduate women. *Child Abuse and Neglect, 25,* 1343–1361.

Gibson, L. E., & Leitenberg, H. (2001). The impact of child sexual abuse and stigma on methods of coping with sexual assault among undergraduate women. *Child Abuse and Neglect, 25,* 1343–1361.

Himelein, M., & McElrath A. (1996). Resilient child sexual abuse survivors: Cognitive coping and illusion. *Child Abuse and Neglect, 20,* 747–758.

Horowitz, A. V., Widom, C. S., McLaughlin, J., & White, H. R. (2001). The impact on childhood abuse and neglect on adult mental health: A prospective study. *Journal of Health and Social Behavior, 42,* 184–201.

Humphrey, J. A., & White, J. W. (2000). Women's vulnerability to sexual assault from adolescence to young adulthood. *Journal of Adolescent Health, 27,* 419–424.

Hyun, M. Friedman, S. D., & Dunner, D. L. (2000). Relationship of childhood physical and sexual abuse to adult bipolar disorder. *Bipolar Disorders, 2,* 131–135.

Kendall-Tackett, K. A., Williams, L. M., & Finkelhor, D. (1993). Impact of sexual abuse on children: A review and synthesis of recent empirical studies. *Psychological Bulletin, 113,* 164–180.

Kendler, K. S., Bulik, C. M., Silberg J., Hettema J. M., Myers, J., & Prescott C. A. (2000). Childhood sexual abuse and adult psychiatric and substance abuse disorders in women. *Archives of General Psychiatry, 57,* 953–959.

Koverola, C., & Foy, D. (1993). Post traumatic stress disorder symptomatology in sexual abused children: Implications for legal proceedings. *Journal of Child Sexual Abuse, 2,* 119–128.

Kristensen, E., & Lau, M. (2007). Women with a history of childhood sexual abuse: Long-term social and psychiatric aspects. *Nordic Journal of Psychiatry, 61,* 115–120.

Landecker, H. (1992). The role of childhood sexual trauma in the etiology of borderline personality disorder: Considerations for diagnosis and treatment. *Psychotherapy, 29,* 234–242.

Lemieux, S. R., & Byers, E. S. (2008). The sexual well-being of women who have experienced child sexual abuse. *Psychology of Women Quarterly, 32,* 126–144.

Liem, J. H., O'Toole, J. G., & James, J. B. (1992). The need for power in women who were sexually abused as children: An exploratory study. *Psychology of Women Quarterly, 16,* 467–480.

Lundberg-Love, P. K. (1990). Adult survivors of incest. In R. T. Ammerman and M. Hersen (Eds.), *Treatment of family violence: A sourcebook* (pp. 211–240). New York: Wiley.

Lundberg-Love, P. K. (1999). The resilience of the human psyche: Recognition and treatment of the adult incest survivor. In M. A. Paludi (Ed.), *The psychology of sexual victimization: A handbook* (pp. 3–30). Westport, CT: Greenwood.

McDonagh, A., McHugo, G., Sengupta, A., Demment, C. C., Schnurr, P. P., Friedman, M., Ford, J., Meuser, K., Fournier, D., & Descamps, M. (2005). Randomized trial of cognitive-behavioral therapy for chronic post-traumatic stress disorder in adult female survivors of childhood sexual abuse. *Journal of Consulting and Clinical Psychology, 73,* 515–524.

McLeer, S. V., Deblinger, E., Atkins, M. S., Foa, E. B., & Ralphe, D. L. (1988). Post-traumatic stress disorder in sexually abused children. *Journal of the American Academy of Child and Adolescent Psychiatry, 27,* 650–654.

McMullin, D., Wirth, R. J., & White, J. W. (2007). The impact of sexual victimization on personality: A longitudinal study of gendered attributes. *Sex Roles, 56,* 403–414.

McNally, R. J. (1993). Stressors that produce post-traumatic stress disorder in children. In J. R. T. Davison & E. G. Foa (Eds.), *Post-traumatic stress disorder: DSM-IV and beyond* (pp. 57–74). Washington, DC: American Psychiatric Press.

Molnar, B. E., Buka, S. L., & Kessler, R. C. (2001). Child sexual abuse and subsequent psychopathology: Results from the National Comorbidity Survey. *American Journal Public Heath, 91,* 743–760.

Mulder, R., Beautrais, A., Joyce, P., & Fergusson, D. (1998). Relationship between dissociation, childhood sexual abuse, childhood physical abuse, and mental illness in a general population sample. *American Journal of Psychiatry, 155,* 806–811.

Nelson, S. (2002). Physical symptoms in sexually abused women: Somatization or undetected injury? *Child Abuse Review, 11,* 51–64.

Putman, S. E. (2009). The monsters in my head: Post-traumatic stress disorder and the child survivor of sexual abuse. *Journal of Counseling & Development, 87,* 80–89.

Rich, C. L., Combs-Lane, A. M., Resnick, H. S., & Kilpatrick, D. G. (2004). Child sexual abuse and adult sexual revictimization. In L. J. Koenig, L. S. Doll, A. O'Leary, and W. Pequegnant (Eds.), *Child sexual abuse to adult sexual risk: Trauma, revictimization, and intervention* (pp. 49–68). Washington, DC: American Psychological Association.

Roosa, M. W., Reyes, L., Reinholtz, C., & Angelini, P. J. (1998). Measurement of women's child sexual abuse experiences: An empirical demonstration of the impact of choice of measure on estimates of incidence rates and of relationships with pathology. *Journal of Sex Research, 35,* 225–233.

Rowan, A. B., & Foy, D. W. (1993). Post-traumatic stress disorder in child sexual abuse survivors: A literature review. *Journal of Traumatic Stress, 6,* 3–20.

Siegler, R., DeLoache, J., & Eisenberg, N. (2003). *How children develop.* New York: Worth Publishers.

Terr, L. C. (1989). *A proposal for an overall DSM-IV category, post traumatic stress.* Paper prepared for the DSM-IV Work Group on Post-traumatic Stress Disorder.

United States Census Bureau (2008). *Annual estimates of the resident population by sex and five-year age groups for the United States: April 1, 2000 to July 1, 2008.*

Retrieved on September 20, 2010, from http://www.census.gov/popest/national/asrh/NC-EST2008-sa.html.

United States Department of Health and Human Services (2008). *What is child abuse and neglect?* Washington, DC: U.S. Government Printing Office.

United States Department of Health and Human Services (2010). *Child Maltreatment 2010.* Washington, DC: U.S. Government Printing Office.

Walker, J. L., Carey, P. D., Mohr, N., Stein, D. J., & Seedat, S. (2004). Gender differences in the prevalence of childhood sexual abuse and in the development of pediatric PTSD. *Archives of Womens Mental Health, 7,* 111–121.

Walsh, K., Blaustein, M., Knight, W. G., Spinazzola, J., & van der Kolk, B. A. (2007). Resiliency factors in the relation between childhood sexual abuse and adult sexual assault in college-age women. *Journal of Child Sexual Abuse, 16,* 1–17.

Wyatt, G. E., & Peters, S. D. (1986). Issues in the definition of child sexual abuse in prevalence research. *Child Abuse and Neglect, 10,* 231–240.

Chapter 3

Women Diagnosed with HIV/AIDS

Experiences of Abuse, Victimization, and Discrimination

Julie Ramos and Kevin L. Nadal

CASE STUDY

Janet Rodriguez (pseudonym) is a 40-year-old Latina woman who is currently a patient at a facility that specializes in helping women who have been infected with HIV/AIDS. Janet receives individual counseling and also attends group therapy once a week. She has been living with HIV for more than 20 years, and although she has accepted her diagnosis, she struggles every day with the various traumas that she has endured throughout her life.

Janet admits to having a troubled childhood. Her father was an alcoholic, and she was neglected by her mother emotionally and physically. Janet's living situation with her parents became so unbearable that she was sent to live with her maternal grandparents when she was a toddler. However, while she was living there she was sexually molested repeatedly by both of these grandparents, leading to further mistrust in her family members and adults in general. Furthermore, when Janet was only 8 years old she was kidnapped off the street by three men who repeatedly raped, sodomized, and beat her for hours. They left her torn and broken body in a basement, not knowing whether or not she was still alive. Luckily a neighbor heard her cries, and she was taken to the hospital in time. While she survived the incident, she developed an intense fear of the dark (nyctophobia) as well as a fear of being on subway trains or in other confined spaces for extended periods of time (claustrophobia). Janet repressed the traumatic memory for years, which enabled the phobias to continue.

When Janet became a young woman, her life spiraled out of control as she jumped from one dysfunctional or abusive relationship to the other. She eventually had three children, from different fathers, and was often the victim of domestic violence in each of these relationships. Because of the unsafe environments that she lived in, all three of her children were taken away by Child Protective Services. Janet then became addicted to crack, heroin, and marijuana. She even began to sell her body to support her drug habits. Eventually Janet discovered that she was HIV-positive. When she was first diagnosed with the disease, she had no idea if she had contracted it from her drug use, her sexual encounters, or some combination of both.

Sadly, Janet's story is not so different than the stories of a lot of the other women who have come to the facility for counseling. A large number of these patients reported histories of childhood sexual abuse, physical victimization and assault, and neglect. A number of the women have engaged in unprotected sex while under the influence of drugs. Many women sold their bodies to support their drug habits, and many mothers have lost custody of their children. Despite the myriad experiences that eventually brought these women to seek treatment, the common denominator among all of them is that they have been diagnosed with HIV/AIDS.

It is true that today being diagnosed as HIV-positive is no longer considered a death sentence. However, there is a still a strong stigma associated with the disease, particularly for women. Women who are diagnosed with HIV/AIDS experience a number of issues, including the responsibility of keeping themselves healthy, of breaking the news to their families if they choose to do so, and perhaps of taking care of their children. The purpose of the current chapter is to examine the literature involving women who have been diagnosed with HIV/AIDS. The chapter will explore the common experiences of victimization and abuse that many of these women have encountered throughout their lives. The chapter will then review the types of discrimination and stigma that these women experience because of their HIV status. Finally, the chapter will provide recommendations for providing the most effective counseling and psychotherapy for women who are HIV-positive, highlighting elements that clinicians should be aware of when working with this population.

WOMEN WITH HIV/AIDS AND HISTORIES OF ABUSE OR VICTIMIZATION

In recent years there has been an increase in literature focusing on the relationship between childhood sexual abuse and women who have been diagnosed as HIV-positive (Evans et al., 1997). Browne and Finkelhor (1986) found that women who experience childhood sexual, physical, or emotional abuse are especially at risk for psychological difficulties, namely depression, anxiety, and substance abuse problems. Women who suffer from these mental health issues may often engage in riskier sexual behaviors and more problematic substance use, making them more susceptible to contracting HIV/AIDS. Messman-Moore and Long (2000) found that women who experienced childhood sexual abuse or adult sexual assault were often revictimized, leading to the development of avoidant coping strategies (e.g., substance abuse, unprotected sex). Finally, Simoni and Ng (2000) found that 230 women living with HIV/AIDS in New York City had high rates of physical or sexual abuse in childhood (50%) and adulthood (68%) and that 7% of these women had also been raped or physically assaulted in the last 90 days.

These studies and others indicate that there is a pattern of early childhood abuse and later HIV infection. Wyatt et al. (2002) found that women who report early and chronic sexual abuse are seven times more likely to engage in HIV-related high-risk behaviors. The same study also reported that women who are HIV-positive have more sexual partners, more sexually transmitted diseases, and more severe histories of abuse than HIV-negative women. Furthermore, sexual abuse, incidents of attempted and completed rape, and physical abuse in childhood put women at an increased risk for HIV infection, and African American women who were HIV-positive had a higher likelihood of reporting histories of child abuse that put them at an increased risk for engaging in sexual behaviors that may have caused their illnesses (Wyatt et al., 2002).

Previous research has also indicated that histories of childhood abuse may also impact medication compliance and treatment. A study by Liu et al. (2006) reported that there may be aspects of a woman's early sexual abuse experiences and current environment that may influence substance abuse, psychological vulnerability, and medication adherence. The study found that unemployment, economic disadvantages, depression, drugs, social isolation, and lack of education were common factors that affected medication compliance for women with histories of childhood abuse. Finally, participants who abused harder drugs and who had lower self-esteem were less likely to adhere to medication. Again, because these women had suffered from childhood abuse, they developed faulty coping mechanisms, which then led to riskier behaviors and eventually may have led to them contracting HIV.

Myers et al. (2006) investigated how one's childhood sexual abuse impacted HIV-positive women by examining the severity of abuse experiences and the effectiveness of HIV risk and harm reduction interventions. Researchers also explored four major outcomes that are often related with childhood abuse, including (1) risky sexual behavior, (2) severity of post-traumatic stress disorder (PTSD) symptoms, (3) sexual trauma symptoms, and (4) depression. Results found that women who are HIV-positive and have histories of childhood sexual abuse have a higher likelihood of engaging in risky sexual behaviors that either may have contributed to their diagnosis or may be further complicating their health while infected with HIV. Some of these risky sexual behaviors include lower condom use, and more exposure to sexually transmitted diseases.

According to Putnam (2003), women who are abused by family members are associated with more severe PTSD symptoms and revictimization as adults because of the fact that intrafamilial abuse may be more psychologically debilitating. When a child is abused (particularly sexually abused) by a family member, the psychological effects may be compounded for many reasons. First, the betrayal of trust by a family member may result in distrust in all other people, leading to dysfunctional romantic and intimate relationships. Second, when a child is abused by a family member, it is likely for the abusive incidents to persist over a longer period of time. Furthermore, some women who experience several incidents of childhood sexual abuse by a number of different perpetrators (and who experience subsequent sexual abuse or assault in their adult years) may experience profound psychological distress that complicates the women's HIV prevention and treatment (Myers et al., 2006).

Finally, understanding childhood sexual abuse is crucial because some studies have found that when patients with HIV/AIDS also have histories of traumatic events, the progression of their disease tends to be faster than for those without histories of trauma. Kimerling, Armistead, and Forehand (1999) found that experiencing a traumatic event (e.g., rape, assault), particularly when a woman reported PTSD symptoms, led to a significant decrease in helper T-cells than for those who did not experience a traumatic event. Conversely, Antoni et al. (2008) found that providing skills for stress management to HIV-positive women led to a reduction in the likelihood of HIV-related illness, including cervical neoplasia. Thus, not only are HIV-positive women with histories of trauma more susceptible to the progression of HIV/AIDS, but those who receive treatment (i.e., learn to cope with their psychological stressors) may be more likely to decrease their symptoms.

WOMEN WITH HIV/AIDS AND EXPERIENCES WITH DISCRIMINATION

While there is stigma associated with anyone who is diagnosed with HIV, there is even more stigma for women with the disease. Wingood et al. (2007) examined the types of discrimination that women with HIV/AIDS faced. In a study of 366 women with HIV/AIDS in Georgia and Alabama, one-sixth of the sample reported experiencing discrimination due to their HIV status. Women who reported HIV discrimination also reported higher stress levels, suicidal ideation, and depressive symptoms and a higher number of unprotected sexual episodes. Moreover, those who reported discrimination also reported lower mean scores for self-esteem and quality of life and were less likely to seek medical care for their disease. Furthermore, African American women who reported HIV discrimination also reported more severe mental health problems than their White counterparts, suggesting that race is an additional factor that impacts discrimination for women with HIV/AIDS.

Carvalhal (2010) further supports the notion that women with HIV experience a number of challenges that are unique to their population. First, despite the fact that women constitute 50% of HIV/AIDS-related cases, they are among the least studied groups in HIV/AIDS-related research. Second, because of their gender, women with HIV/AIDS experience stigma and discrimination due to gendered social and work roles that men do not hold. Third, in addition to the psychological problems that these women often endure, many of them report a lack of access to health care, financial assistance, emotional and social support, and family services. Parents with HIV/AIDS often experience a number of problems with poor housing and unsafe neighborhoods. Finally, women with HIV/AIDS often experience stigma, discrimination, racism, and poverty as a result of their disease.

Race also plays an important factor for women who are diagnosed with HIV/AIDS. Women of color, particularly African American and Latina women, tend to be diagnosed at much higher rates than their White female counterparts. While African American and Latina women together represent 12% of all women in the United States, they account for more than 61% of all new HIV infections (Prejean, Song, An, & Hall, 2008). Furthermore, HIV/AIDS was the third leading cause of death for African American women ages 25 to 34 in 2006 (National Center for Injury Prevention and Control, 2009). Because women of color are likely to be discriminated against on the basis of their race, gender, or some combination of both, those who are diagnosed with HIV/AIDS face further discrimination from those in the general community as well as from those in their own racial or ethnic communities. Women of color who are also of lower socioeconomic statuses bear an additional burden of overcoming all sorts of discrimination while also coping with financial burdens (particularly financial burdens that are caused by their illness).

COUNSELING WOMEN WITH HIV/AIDS

Clinicians who have female clients who are HIV-positive have an added responsibility in their profession. Counselors must be aware of the research on this population and also familiarize themselves with the illness itself in order to be most effective in working with their clients. Previous literature has discussed a variety of issues concerning female clients who are HIV-positive. For instance, it has been found that most HIV/AIDS prevention programs address only consensual sexual practices and fail to address the psychological consequences of early childhood abuse on sexual decision making (Wyatt et al., 2002). If prevention programs neglect to address the issue of early abuse and its link to HIV/AIDS, the assumption can be made that those who are already infected may not be receiving the additional psychological care that they require. Therefore, counselors and clinicians should be aware of the possible link between abuse and HIV/AIDS, cautiously inquiring about the possibility of such histories. In cases where there are histories of abuse or victimization, it would be helpful for clinicians to address the traumas directly in order to confront one potential source of their clients' presenting problems.

Counselors and clinicians may also benefit from knowing how these women cope with their illness as well as the ways that they have coped with their stressors throughout their lives. According to Simoni and Ng (2000), an important determinant of psychological adaptation to trauma is the way in which an individual copes with that experience. Women who utilize problem-focused strategies (e.g., rational actions, help-seeking behaviors, cognitive restructuring, and religious activities) have been found to show lower levels of psychological distress; meanwhile, women who utilize negative coping strategies (e.g., denial and avoidance) show greater psychological distress, which is evident in childhood sexual abuse survivors (Simoni & Ng, 2000). It has also been found that HIV-infected women use avoidant strategies to cope with their illness, perhaps due to diminished hopes of recovery as their disease progresses over time (Simoni & Ng, 2000). Thus, it is important for clinicians to be cognizant of women's faulty coping mechanisms and to promote healthier ways for women to manage their psychological stressors.

Previous literature has also reported that women who blamed themselves for their HIV diagnosis also had high levels of emotional and psychological distress (Simoni & Ng, 2000). When an individual first learns of her HIV/AIDS status, she may feel a great deal of regret and shame. Thus, one goal in psychotherapy would be to assist a client in grieving the loss of her HIV-negative status. Similar to other forms of grief (e.g., death of a loved one, acceptance of a terminal illness), an individual may experience a number of stages in coping with her loss. For example, it may be common for individuals to initially deal with denial, anger, bargaining, and sadness while eventually learning to accept their status.

Regarding ethnicity, African American women were more likely to report to the counselor that they felt responsible for their illness and were more likely to internalize their feelings when compared to White women and Latina women, who were more likely to use praying, daydreaming, and drug use to cope with their HIV status (Simoni & Ng, 2000). Moreover, counselors should work to develop a trustful rapport with these clients by approaching the topic in a nonjudgmental manner so that clients may effectively reveal accounts of trauma, and counselors must also be able to recognize signs of abuse in order to refer clients to more experienced clinicians if need be (Simoni & Ng, 2000). Mental health professionals must be willing to pay greater attention to childhood abuse instead of adopting the tendency of focusing on the immediate presenting problem, because research has shown that women's current functioning is greatly impacted by the effects of that early trauma even more so than from a recent trauma (Herman, 1992).

According to Myers et al. (2006), current efforts to reduce HIV transmission and to counsel those already infected are lacking because they sometimes neglect to focus on the cumulative psychological burden of childhood sexual abuse. In other words, clients are not confronting their initial traumas, possible revictimization, and possible drug use, which may then lead to ineffective mental health treatment. Furthermore, because of their diagnosis, their history of abuse, and other life stressors, women with HIV/AIDS are also at an increased risk for suicidal ideation (Cooperman & Simoni, 2005). While motherhood and spirituality may be protective factors against suicide, it has also been found that women with HIV/AIDS had an increase in suicide attempts on the first anniversary of their diagnosis (Cooperman & Simoni, 2005). Thus, it is crucial for women who are diagnosed with HIV/AIDS to seek counseling immediately in order to minimize their likelihood for suicide ideation.

For women who have been infected with HIV/AIDS, disclosure is another topic that may be broached in the psychotherapeutic relationship. According to Leonard and Ellen (2008), disclosure of HIV/AIDS is thought of as a breaking point and is only possible when the client has come to accept her diagnosis and is ready to integrate that illness into her life. Women who are diagnosed with HIV/AIDS may be fearful of disclosing their status because they may have already experienced forced sex with an infected person, unprotected sex due to fear of abuse, or domestic violence, which may make them hesitant to label themselves with the illness (Gielen, McDonnell, O'Campo, & Burke, 2005). These women could possibly fear that their families or significant others may ostracize them or become violent with them, or such women could be afraid of how their HIV status will affect their relationships with their loved ones. There may be shame in admitting that they contracted the disease through unprotected sex or drug use. Thus, a major initial focus of counseling or psychotherapy would be for a client to come to terms with the disease and learn to feel comfortable in disclosing her status to her loved ones.

When women with HIV/AIDS do seek mental health treatment, they may even experience stigma or discrimination from their therapists. Roberts, Grusky, and Swanson (2008) aimed to uncover the perceptions of HIV test counselors by examining individuals' experiences with a variety of "difficult" and "good" clients. Results indicate that a number of factors contribute to how clients are labeled, including patients' actual characteristics, HIV test counselor characteristics, and HIV testing environments, suggesting that clinicians should be aware of their own biases in working with HIV-positive women and not let those biases impact the relationship. Counselors may respond to clients whom they label as "difficult" in a negative fashion, thus neglecting to provide the adequate care that they deserve. Ultimately it is important that for mental health practitioners to treat their clients with the utmost respect, recognizing that all of their clients may have both good and difficult days. When necessary, Roberts, Grusky, and Swanson argue that clinicians should confer with other mental health professionals when dealing with difficult clients and refer such patients when they recognize that alternative treatment would be more effective.

In conclusion, providing mental health treatment for women with HIV is a daunting task because of the cumulative nature of all of the dynamics that are involved. Childhood abuse histories, substance abuse history, current victimization and assault, and even multicultural issues should be taken into consideration when working with this population. A number of women with HIV/AIDS are also dealing with dual traumas or diagnoses such as substance abuse, domestic violence, poverty, inadequate housing, and a chaotic life overall, which puts them at a huge risk for further mental health issues (Tarakeshwar, Fox, Ferro, Khawaja, & Kochman, 2005). Furthermore, as discussed throughout the chapter, coping with childhood sexual abuse or adult victimization are two major factors that may exacerbate the effects of women's HIV/AIDS diagnoses, especially if they have not yet confronted their initial traumas. For counselors and therapists, having an understanding of the nature of past experiences can help in designing interventions that will effectively address the specific needs of women who are HIV-positive (Myers et al., 2006).

At the same time, clinicians must be aware that each HIV/AIDS case is different. Not all women with HIV/AIDS have histories of childhood abuse or victimization. Not all women with HIV/AIDS have histories of substance abuse or risky sexual behavior. In fact, women who fit the opposite of this profile are also susceptible to contracting the disease, particularly if they engage in unsafe sex. Thus, it is the role of mental health practitioners to provide the most effective treatment for all clients, taking into consideration how women's personal experiences, identities, and worldviews may affect how they cope with their HIV/AIDS status and how their status affects their mental health, psychological processes, and self-esteem.

REFERENCES

Antoni, M. H., Pereira, D. B., Marion, I., Ennis, N., Andrasik, M. P., Rose, R., Lucci, J. (2008). Stress management effects on perceived stress and cervical neoplasia in low-income HIV-infected women. *Journal of Psychosomatic Research, 65,* 389–401.

Browne, A., & Finkelhor, D. (1986). Impact of childhood sexual abuse: A Review of the research. *Psychological Bulletin, 99,* 66–77.

Carvalhal, A. (2010). Are women a different group of HIV-infected individuals? *Archives of Women's Mental Health, 13,* 181–183.

Cooperman, N., & Simoni, J. (2005). Suicidal ideation and attempted suicide among women living with HIV/AIDS. *Journal of Behavioral Medicine, 28,* 149–156.

Evans, D., Leserman, J., Perkins, D., Stern, R., Murphy, C., Zheng, B., & Petitto, J. M. (1997). Severe life stress as a predictor of early disease progression in HIV infection. *American Journal of Psychiatry, 154,* 630–634.

Gielen, A. C., McDonnell, K., O'Campo, P., & Burke, J. (2005). Suicide risk and mental health indicators: Do they differ by abuse and HIV status? *Women's Health Issues, 15,* 89–95.

Herman, J. L. (1992). *Trauma and recovery.* New York: Basic Books.

Kimerling, R., Armistead, L., & Forehand, R. (1999). Victimization experiences and HIV infected women: Associations with serostatus, psychological symptoms, and health status. *Journal of Traumatic Stress, 12,* 41–58.

Leonard, L., & Ellen, J. (2008). The story of my life: AIDS and autobiographical occasions. *Qualitative Sociology, 31,* 37–56.

Leserman, J., Drossman, D. A., Li, Z., Toomey, T. C., Nachman, G., & Glogau, L. (1996). Sexual and physical abuse in gastroenterology practice: How types of abuse impact health status. *Psychosomatic Medicine, 58,* 4–15.

Liu, H., Longshore, D., Williams, J., Rivkin, I., Loeb, T., Warda, U., Carmona, J., & Wyatt, G. (2006). Substance abuse and medication adherence among HIV positive women with histories of child sexual abuse. *AIDS and Behavior, 10,* 279–286.

Messman-Moore, T. L., & Long, P. J. (2000). The revictimization of childhood sexual abuse survivors: An examination of the adjustment of college women with child sexual abuse, adult sexual assault, and adult physical abuse. *Child Maltreatment, 5,* 18–27.

Myers, H., Wyatt, G., Burns, T., Carmona, J., Warda, U., Longshore, D., Rivkin, I., Chin, D., & Liu, H. (2006). Severity of child sexual abuse, post-traumatic stress, and risky sexual behaviors among HIV positive women. *AIDS and Behavior, 10,* 191–198.

National Center for Injury Prevention and Control. (2009). WISQARS leading causes of death reports. Retrieved on February 3, 2011, from http://webappa.cdc.gov/sasweb/ncipc/leadcaus10.html.

Prejean, J., Song, R., An, Q., & Hall, H. (2008). *Subpopulation estimates from the HIV Incidence Surveillance System—United States, 2006.* Division of HIV/AIDS Prevention, National Center for HIV/AIDS, Viral Hepatitis, STD, and TB Prevention, Centers for Disease Control and Prevention. Retrieved on February 3, 2011, from http://www.cdc.gov/mmwr/preview/mmwrhtml/mm5736a1.htm.

Putnam, F. (2003). Ten-year research update review: Child sexual abuse. *Journal of the American Academy of Child and Adolescent Psychiatry, 42,* 269–278.

Roberts, K. J., Grusky, O., & Swanson, A. N. (2008). Client encounters in alternative HIV testing sites: Counselors' perceptions and experiences. *Behavioral Medicine, 34,* 11–18.

Rose, R. C., House, A. S., Stepleman, L. M. (2010). Intimate partner violence and its effects on the health of African American HIV-positive women. *Psychological Trauma: Theory, Research, Practice, and Policy, 2,* 311–317.

Simoni, J. M., & Ng, M. T. (2000). Trauma, coping, and depression among women with HIV/AIDS in New York City. *AIDS Care, 12,* 567–580.

Tarakeshwar, N., Fox, A., Ferro, C., Khawaja, S., & Kochman, A. (2005). The connections between childhood sexual abuse and human immunodeficiency virus infection implications for interventions. *Journal of Community Psychology, 33,* 655–672.

Wingood, G. M., Hardin, J. W., DiClemente, R. J., Peterson, S. H., Mikhail, I., Hook, E. W., McCree, D. H., Saag, M., Davies, S. L. (2007). HIV discrimination and the health of women living with HIV. *Women & Health, 46,* 99–112.

Wyatt, G., Myers, H., Williams, J., Kitchen, C. R., Loeb, T., Carmona, J., Wyatt, L., Chin, D., & Presley, N. (2002). Does a history of trauma contribute to HIV risk for women of color? Implications for prevention and policy. *American Journal of Public Health, 92,* 660–665.

Chapter 4

Verbal Sexual Coercion in Young Adult Heterosexual Dating Relationships

Jennifer Katz, Vanessa Tirone, and Melanie Schukrafft

> It was my boyfriend at the time and I did not realize I was being emotionally abused. I was never physically forced in any way and so at the time never considered it an issue.

> I wasn't ever "raped" per se, and he was my boyfriend of over a year. He pressured me and told me how important sex in our relationship was to him and it made me feel guilty for not wanting to always have sex with him, so I would have intercourse even if I didn't want to.

> I was not actually raped and I didn't consider the guy to be particularly dangerous because we had been casually dating when he pressured me to be in a more physical relationship.

> He was my boyfriend and it didn't seem like it was a big deal. He just begged all the time for it so I gave in even though I didn't really want it.

This chapter reviews theory and research related to verbal sexual coercion in young adult heterosexual dating relationships. We opened with just a few student responses to an anonymous campus-wide survey at a small public college. Students were asked about their nonconsensual sexual experiences and about obstacles to reporting these experiences to campus personnel. In response, many students described being verbally coerced into unwanted sex by dating partners. These representative quotes illustrate both the construct of verbal sexual coercion and some reasons why it is controversial.

Verbal sexual coercion is often viewed as socially acceptable, particularly within dating relationships. It is not illegal or criminal to verbally coerce sex from an unwilling partner; such behavior is treated as persuasion (McGregor, 2005). Even rape, which is legally recognized and arguably the most serious sexual violation, is often accepted in many situations involving romantic or sexual partners (Muehlenhard & Peterson, 2004). In part this is because sexual violations are viewed differently from other types of violations, such as those involving property rights. Highly personal and diverse attitudes and beliefs about gender and sexuality affect how each of us thinks about sexual violations. Furthermore, consent, resistance, intimidation, and force are conceptualized differently by individuals and from the perspective of the victim ("I didn't say 'yes'") versus perpetrator ("She/He didn't say 'no'"). If a man sexually penetrates an immobile crying woman, has she consented? Does it matter why she is crying? If a woman fellates a sleeping man who previously consented to fellatio, is it rape? If a person follows instructions to undress, however reluctantly, is she or he agreeing to and therefore culpable for what happens next? Such questions become even more contentious when considering sex that is coerced via psychological pressure, rather than via physical force or incapacitation, within dating relationships.

This chapter has three parts. In the first section we define verbal sexual coercion and describe how it is both similar to and yet also different from rape. In the second section we describe typical operational definitions and the prevalence of verbal sexual coercion in dating samples of young adults. In the third section we discuss sociocultural norms about gender, heterosexuality, and sexual consent in intimate relationships that help to explain how and why verbal sexual coercion occurs in young heterosexual couples. We conclude by challenging common victim-blaming attitudes about women and men who are verbally coerced into sex.

COMPARING VERBAL SEXUAL COERCION AND RAPE

Although verbal sexual coercion is a distinct type of sexual violation, it shares several common features with rape (DeGue & DeLillo, 2004). Like rape, verbal sexual coercion involves nonconsensual penetration of the mouth, vagina, or anus. Unlike rape, verbal sexual coercion occurs when a person is compelled into sexual penetration due to immediate psychological pressure (rather than physical force or incapacitation). Demands made by the coercive partner are overwhelming; it may be easier or safer to give in, especially when a coercive partner persistently ignores a victim's repeated sexual refusals. The verbal tactics used to coerce sex are numerous and may involve intimidation, threats of nonphysical harm (such as to one's reputation or to the relationship), put-downs, swearing, or guilt induction (e.g., Livingston, Buddie, Testa, & VanZile-Tamsen, 2004). Although victims of coerced sex are not physically forced or incapacitated, they are constrained by psychological pressure exerted by the partner in the immediate situation. Verbal sexual coercion is sometimes included when researchers collapse different types of nonviolent sexual violations into such categories as "sexual coercion" (DeGue & DeLillo, 2004) or "nonagentic sexual experiences" (Crown & Roberts, 2007). Other authors have referred to verbal coercion as "heterosexual coercion" (Gavey, 2005) and "interpersonal coercion" (Finklehor & Yllo, 1987) to emphasize that the pressure is psychological in nature.

Like rape, verbal sexual coercion violates individual sexual autonomy. Sexual autonomy includes the right to refuse sexual activity with any person at any time for any or no reason (Schulhofer, 1998). Sexual autonomy is not a legally protected right. In contrast, property laws protect us from threats of slander (extortion), stealth (larceny), or false persuasion (fraud). Schulhofer critiques the focus on physical violence as the standard typically used in legal treatments of rape: "rather than asking whether certain sexual advances unjustifiably impair freedom of choice, we have asked only whether the conduct is so bad that it is equivalent to violent compulsion" (p. 102). The fact that sexual autonomy is not protected in state law (McGregor, 2005) both reflects and corroborates sociocultural tendencies to emphasize the role of victims rather than perpetrators in understanding sexual violations.

Sexual violations, including rape and verbal sexual coercion, are nonconsensual. Sexual consent, as defined here, involves the ability to freely decide whether to be involved in sexual penetration (McGregor, 2005). In cases of verbal coercion, autonomous sexual decision making is constrained by a partner's use of external and immediate psychological pressure. In other words, we argue that surrender or capitulation due to partner pressure does not constitute free and willing consent. At the same time, conditions of free and willing consent are not easily defined, and sexual consent itself is often defined differently by various researchers and individuals (Beres, 2007). Some even define sexual consent as any agreement involving sexual activity regardless of the circumstances. For example, Beres described a case in which a rape victim pleaded with a perpetrator (armed with a knife) to use a condom; the victim's attempt to protect her sexual health was perceived by the court as consent to engage in sex more generally.

Despite varying definitions of sexual consent, it is important to note that consent among adults (in the United States, defined by each state) is presumed unless there is sufficient evidence to the contrary. In other words, the default legal position is that sexual consent exists, a striking presumption "without analogy in law" (McGregor, 2005, p. 104). Consider, for example, medical consent. In general if a physician does not receive explicit permission from patients or their families to medically intervene, the physician may not intervene. This is true even when the physician judges that such procedures would be in a patient's best interests. Laws requiring medical consent exist because we value the right to decide for ourselves what happens to our own bodies. Therefore, nonconsent is the general default position that reflects our right to self-determination. Unlike the gender-neutral laws governing medical practice, however, laws governing sexual violations were originally created to protect male perpetrators from accusations by female victims (McGregor, 2005). Consequently, laws today privilege sexually coercive perpetrators (regardless of their gender) over their victims.

Both rape and verbal sexual coercion frequently evoke victim-blaming responses. The presumption of consent focuses attention on how a victim, rather than a perpetrator, acted (i.e., she/he "stopped saying no," "said no but didn't mean it," "eventually stopped saying no," "was silent," "didn't push me away"). Because of this focus, victim behavior, appearance, or other characteristics are common grounds for minimizing sexual violations or even dismissing legal charges; in contrast, victims of theft or fraud are permitted to engage in potentially inadvisable behaviors. For example, if a woman invites her date home and this person steals her stereo equipment, she is not seen as having consented. Another reason for victim blaming is that perpetrators are often seen as lacking self-control over their own libidinal desires. Ironically enough, this perception shifts responsibility to the person whose behavior was unconstrained by apparently overwhelming sexual passion: the victim (Anderson & Doherty, 2008).

Most sexual violations, including rape and verbal sexual coercion, are perpetrated by men against women (Bourke, 2007). In fact, more heterosexual men perpetrate sexually coercive acts than either heterosexual women or sexual minorities of either gender (VanderLaan & Vasey, 2009). Accordingly, most of the research that we review involves male perpetration and female victimization. At the same time, boys and men can and do experience sexual violations perpetrated by girls and women, and this is especially clear when considering verbal sexual coercion specifically. Dismissing or minimizing male victimization by women both trivializes the experiences of male victims and perpetuates mistaken stereotypes about powerless females and inviolable males (Bourke, 2007; Gavey, 2005).

Like rape, verbal sexual coercion involves nonconsensual penetration, violates sexual autonomy, commonly evokes victim blaming, and disproportionately affects girls and women. Despite these commonalities, rape and verbal sexual coercion differ in important ways. For example, compared to women who have experienced forcible rape or rape due to intoxication, women are more likely to attribute episodes of verbal sexual coercion as due at least partly to miscommunication (Abbey, BeShears, Clinton-Sherrod, & McAuslan, 2004). In addition, low assertiveness is a predictor of women's verbal sexual coercion but not of rape (Testa & Derman, 1999). Although rates of forced sex in heterosexual relationships are low among dating men as compared to dating women (e.g., Slashinski, Coker, & Davis, 2003), most men who are sexually violated by women experience verbal sexual coercion, not rape (e.g., Struckman-Johnson, 1988). And perhaps most germane to the present chapter, verbal sexual coercion is much more common than rape by intimate partners, who typically can obtain sexual access without using physical force or substances (Abbey et al., 2004; Lyndon, Whitee & Kadlec, 2007). For these reasons, a focus on understanding verbal sexual coercion specifically in dating is warranted.

PREVALENCE OF VERBAL SEXUAL COERCION IN YOUNG ADULT HETEROSEXUAL DATING RELATIONSHIPS

Craig (1990) published a seminal review of sexual coercion, defined broadly, within dating relationships. Since 1990, relatively few studies have documented rates of verbal sexual coercion specifically within young adult heterosexual dating couples. To include as many studies as possible since Craig's review, we defined dating rather broadly to include one-night stands, dates, and longer-lasting relationships excluding cohabitation or marriage. We excluded studies that reported lifetime experiences of verbal sexual coercion that did not necessarily occur in a dating relationship. We also excluded studies that did not specifically assess verbal sexual coercion in a dating relationship even if general sexual coercion in dating was assessed. In contrast, because heterosexual dating is commonly presumed (rather than directly assessed), we included studies of verbal sexual coercion in dating that did not assess the perpetrator's sex (as noted below).

All of the studies that we found were conducted with samples from either high school or college settings; we found no data on verbal sexual coercion among either school dropouts or homeless youths who date, although such populations may be at increased risk for sexual violations generally (e.g., Tyler & Johnson, 2006). Furthermore, many of the studies sample primarily Caucasian middle-class young people in North America, which limits our knowledge about verbal sexual coercion in dating more generally. Based on the available research, we found that many young people experience verbal sexual coercion in dating relationships; at the same time, specific prevalence rates vary across operational definitions and specific samples.

SEXUAL EXPERIENCES SURVEY

The most widely used measure of sexual victimization is the Sexual Experiences Survey (SES) (Koss & Oros, 1982), which has been updated and validated in recent years (e.g., Testa, VanZile-Tamsen, Livingston, & Koss, 2004). Two SES items comprise the sexual coercion subscale; both involve psychological pressure due to either partner authority or continual arguments and pressure. Research using the SES has shown that verbal sexual coercion is a relatively common experience for women in dating relationships. In a study of sexual coercion during dates in college, Patton and Mannison (1995) found that 11% of female college students in their Australian sample (heterosexuality presumed) had been coerced into sex by continual arguments and pressure. Rates appear to be higher in ongoing sexually active relationships. In a sample of U.S. female undergraduates who had consented to sex with their current male dating partner, Katz and Myhr (2008) found that 21% also reported being coerced into sex by the partner's overwhelming continual arguments and pressure.

Rates of sexual coercion reported by men on the SES tend to be lower than rates reported by women. For example, in a sample of American college students,

O'Sullivan, Byers, and Finkelman (1998) reported a significant sex difference; 26% of women and 7% of men reported being verbally coerced into sex in a heterosexual relationship over the past year. Likewise, in another sample of American college students, Harned (2001) found about 13% of women and 8% of men reported being verbally coerced into sex on past dates or in dating relationships (although heterosexuality was presumed, and Harned noted that some of the men's coercion seems to have been perpetrated by other men).

Rates of SES verbal sexual coercion in dating relationships are lower in samples of high school students compared to college. In a sample of American girls about to enter college, Vogel and Himelein (1995) found that about 5% reported being verbally coerced into sex on a date. As in college samples, verbal sexual coercion is more common among girls than boys in high school. For example, in a sample of Canadian high school students with heterosexual dating experience, Poitras and Lavoie (1995) found that 19% of girls and 3% of boys reported having been verbally coerced into sex. Overall, studies using the SES to define verbal sexual coercion suggest that this type of sexual coercion is not uncommon in young adult dating relationships.

REVISED CONFLICT TACTICS SCALES

Another measure commonly used to assess sexual coercion in dating relationships is the Revised Conflict Tactics Scales (CTS2) (Straus, Hamby, Boney-McCoy, & Sugarman, 1996), which includes a seven-item sexual coercion subscale. Sexually coercive tactics are classified as either minor (e.g., "My partner insisted on sex when I did not want to but did not use force") or severe (e.g., "My partner used force, like hitting, holding down, or using a weapon, to make me have sex"). Minor items correspond with a definition of coerced or unprotected sex due to partner verbal sexual coercion, whereas severe items signify physical coercion/rape.

In a sample of unmarried Canadian women who had been in at least one dating relationship lasting at least a month (heterosexuality presumed), about 33% reported that their partners coerced them into sex, yet less than 5% reported any severe (physical) sexual coercion (Brownridge, 2006). Similarly, in a sample of American college women in heterosexual dating relationships, Katz, Kuffel, and Brown (2006) found that 29% endorsed current dating partner sexual coercion on the CTS2; because only 6% endorsed severe coercion, most coercion was due to verbal pressure rather than threatened or actual physical force. Offman and Matheson (2004) found that 18% of their American sample of college women in heterosexual relationships experienced partner sexual coercion on the CTS2 over the past month; presumably most incidents involved verbal pressure based on the findings of both Brownridge (2006) and Katz et al. (2006).

Gender differences in rates of sexual coercion on the CTS2 have been reported inconsistently. In a sample of Polish college students, 57% of women and 38% of men reported partner minor sexual coercion on the CTS2, indicating that a (presumably heterosexual) partner had insisted that they engage in vaginal, anal, oral, or some form of unprotected sexual penetration (Doroszewicz & Forbes, 2008). In contrast, sex differences were not found by Hines (2007), who reported that 25% of women and 22% of men in college (all heterosexual) reported minor sexual coercion over the past year across 32 international sites. However, not all participants were in a dating relationship over the past year, and the gender of the perpetrator was not directly assessed. In addition, Hines and Saudino (2003) suggested previously that women and men may interpret the same items differently, leading to biased estimates. This possibility is also supported by O'Leary and Williams (2006), who found poor within-couple agreement on reports from the CTS2 sexual coercion scale within a sample of American marriages. In addition, because the CTS2 was administered across many countries in different languages, there may also have been cultural differences in item interpretation.

Other research suggests that there may be more reliable sex differences specifically in the frequency of verbal coercion within ongoing heterosexual relationships. Although Kaestle (2009) did not use the CTS2, she found no difference in the proportions of college women and men in heterosexual dating relationships lasting at least three months who had engaged in unwanted sex because their partner insisted on it. However, a significantly greater proportion of these American women (12%) than men (3%) repeatedly experienced coerced sex, often penetration of the mouth or anus. Kaestle's findings match other research using the CTS2. For example, Katz, Carino, and Hilton (2002) sampled American college students who had been in a heterosexual relationship for at least two months; men reported perpetrating significantly more frequent sexual coercion than women, although specific rates were not reported (for sex differences in rates of perpetration in an American dating sample, see also Hines & Saundino, 2003).

Overall, minor sexual coercion on the CTS2, which corresponds to the definition of verbal sexual coercion in this chapter, is common in dating couples worldwide. Relative to studies using the SES, the CTS2 identifies more victims perhaps because it asks about unprotected sex and names different types of sex directly (oral, anal, and vaginal). The larger number of male victims identified may be explained by multiple factors, including a focus on any penetration versus frequency of perpetration, differences in item interpretation and response sets related to sex and culture, and the common presumption of heterosexuality.

OTHER OPERATIONAL DEFINITIONS

In other research that used neither the SES nor the CTS2, researchers often assessed sexual activity or forced sex on dates and then coded the tactics used. In a landmark study of American college students not covered in Craig's (1990) review, Struckman-Johnson (1988) found that 22% of women and 16% of men were forced to have sex on a date (heterosexuality presumed) in their lifetimes. Of those who had experienced forced sex, 55% of women were raped, 19% reported both rape and verbal sexual coercion, and 16% reported verbal coercion only; in contrast,

10% of men were raped, 28% reported both rape and verbal sexual coercion, and 52% reported partner use of verbal coercion only. Similarly, Waldner-Haugrud and Magruder (1995) asked American college students about a range of coercive behaviors "with a date" (heterosexuality presumed) and for each the most extreme outcome (kissing, fondling, intercourse). Women were significantly more likely than men to experience coerced penetration, although rates associated with verbal coercion specifically were not reported. There were sex differences in reports of coercive tactics experienced, although these tactics did not necessarily lead to sexual penetration; women were more likely to experience detainment, lies, and being held down, whereas men were more likely to experience blackmail.

Finally, researchers studying young adults' sexual coercion based on evolutionary theory focus solely on male perpetration and female victimization. Shackelford and Goetz (2004) developed the Sexual Coercion in Intimate Relationships Scale (SCIR) to assess men's sexual coercion of female partners. This scale has three subscales: (a) resource manipulation (e.g., "My partner reminded me of gifts or other benefits he gave me so that I would feel obligated to have sex with him"), (b) commitment manipulation (e.g., "My partner hinted that if I loved him I would have sex with him"), and (c) defection threat (e.g., "My partner hinted that he might pursue a long-term relationship with another woman if I did not have sex with him"). In studies using the SCIR, American college students in dating relationships commonly experienced verbal sexual coercion. For example, 50% of heterosexual women in one sample (Starratt, Goetz, Shackelford, McKibbin, & Stewart-Williams, 2008) reported that their dating partner had engaged in at least one sexually coercive behavior, most commonly commitment manipulation (47%) followed by resource manipulation (22%) and threats of defection (17%). Likewise, Goetz and Shackelford (2009) reported that 32% of heterosexual women in intimate relationships reported on the SCIR some kind of verbally coerced sex with their partner.

In summary, across specific operational definitions and types of school-based convenience samples, many women and men in heterosexual dating relationships are verbally coerced into sex. Rates of coercion tend to be especially high among college students relative to younger adolescents and when definitions of dating include past relationships, dates, longer time intervals, or all of these. Across operational definitions, women are more frequently verbally coerced into sex than men, although men's experiences should not be ignored. Furthermore, presumptions of heterosexuality and the varying cultural contexts require some caution in interpreting some study results.

VERBAL SEXUAL COERCION IN CONTEXT: A BRIEF ANALYSIS OF NORMS RELATED TO GENDER, HETEROSEXUALITY, AND SEXUAL CONSENT IN INTIMATE RELATIONSHIPS

Understanding sexual behavior, including verbal sexual coercion in heterosexual dating relationships, requires consideration of the larger sociocultural context. In this section we consider gendered norms and scripts for young women and men in heterosexual interaction. We also explore normative conceptions of sexual consent in intimate relationships. Because beliefs about race, class, (dis)ability, and other identity categories meaningfully intersect with normative beliefs about gender, heterosexuality, and sexual consent, this discussion is necessarily incomplete. Nonetheless, norms about gender, heterosexuality, and sexual consent have widespread influence. These norms affect how and why verbal sexual coercion occurs, how study participants interpret questions about verbal sexual coercion experiences, and how researchers in this area conduct studies and interpret their data.

Verbal Sexual Coercion and Gender Norms in Heterosexual Context

In Western society, different traits and behaviors are viewed as appropriate for men and women; commonly these behaviors are couched in terms of stereotypical binaries, or opposites (e.g., big/little, competitive/cooperative, dominant/submissive). Through the process of gender socialization, boys and girls learn to behave in ways that are consistent with these gendered expectations, or norms. Although conformity to gender norms is not universal, gender norms are both prescriptive and descriptive. In other words, gender norms influence how people act as well as how they understand themselves and others. Accordingly, the same behaviors enacted by women and men often are evaluated differently because different behaviors are seen as normative and appropriate for each.

Gender norms both reflect and are reflected by common heterosexual mate-selection practices. Boys and men are typically older, taller, and stronger than the girls and women they date. These selection practices promote male power within these relationships and differential risk for female victimization, including verbal sexual coercion. Girls who date older boyfriends are at greater risk for verbal and other forms of sexual coercion than girls who date same-aged peers (Gowen, Feldman, Diaz, & Yisrael, 2004). Given typical gender differences in age, size, and strength within dating couples, many women who are verbally coerced by male partners are psychologically intimidated in ways that some heterosexual men may not readily understand (Muehlenhard & Peterson, 2004).

Gender norms also affect dominant understandings of heterosex (i.e., sex between a man and a woman) and acceptable sexual behaviors for men and women. As described by Holloway (1984), we understand heterosex based on the male sexual drive discourse ("real" men are always eager for sex) and the have/hold discourse (women give sex to men but only in committed relationships for men's pleasure). Consequently, despite individual differences in adherence to these discourses, the same behaviors enacted by young men and women differentially affect their social reputations (Holland, Ramazanoglu, Sharpe, & Thompson, 2004). In public, young men and women presumably have conflicting interests in which men desire sex and women desire love. Appearing to fulfill these desires legitimizes boys as "real men" and girls as "real women" in their peer groups and, by extension, in their own self-views.

Holland et al.'s (2004) extensive interviews with London youths reveal that adolescent males publicly affirm their masculinity by telling stories of sexual conquest; such stories often employ metaphors of battle and conquest, involving, for example, "nailing," "screwing," or "jumping." In doing so, these boys access a public language of sexual agency inappropriate for girls. These narratives imply that a true sexual conquest does not just involve engaging in sex. Rather, conquests involve encountering sexual resistance from a female partner and overcoming that resistance, much like a mugger "jumps" a victim in the street. Verbal sexual coercion represents a common and relatively socially acceptable way to assert such dominance, as shown in the gendered narratives of coercive sex offered by Irish high school students (Hyde, Drennan, Howlett, & Brady, 2008). In reference to the stories shared by high school girls, Hyde et al. note that "the notion that all men want sex and will push for it" was a predominant theme (p. 487).

Gender norms also shape romantic and sexual interactions between women and men, even among those who otherwise are not gender-conforming (Seal & Ehrhardt, 2003). Sexual scripts, or cognitive schema that characterize a sequence of events, allow people to participate in complicated mutually dependent interactions. Traditionally, sexual scripts position men as sexually dominant and women as sexually reticent, submissive, or both (Byers, 1996). Although gendered sexual scripts are evolving and are subject to both developmental and cultural influences (Seal, O'Sullivan, & Ehrhardt, 2007), changes create confusion and uncertainty about expectations during sexual interactions. Consequently, even as people develop more egalitarian gendered attitudes, gender norms continue to constrain sexual interactions, in part because of perceptions about partner script preferences (e.g., Seal & Ehrhardt, 2003). These scripts affect the likelihood of rape (Littleton & Axsom, 2003) and verbal sexual coercion, especially enacted by males against female partners. In fact, VanderLaan and Vasey (2009) found that conformity to sexual scripts best explained heterosexual men's greater use of nonphysical sexual coercion relative to either gay men or women.

In brief, gender norms affect mate-selection practices, understandings of heterosex, and sexual scripts for heterosexual interaction. By extension, gender norms affect how we understand sexual initiations (including verbally coercive initiations) and responses to sexual initiations (including responses to partner coercive behavior). Neither sexual initiations nor responses to such initiations are gender-neutral behaviors.

Sexual Initiation and Coercion

Men's sexual initiations and use of verbal coercion are easily understood based on traditional gendered sexual scripts. When sexual initiations are interpreted in terms of scripts featuring a male (active initiator)/female (passive gatekeeper) binary, men who initiate sex are acting like men, whereas men who refuse sex are acting like women (Gavey, 2005). These sexual scripts, combined with normative expectations about male sexual dominance and sexual desire, may set the stage for men to both initiate sex and persist in attempts to gain sexual access despite a partner's disinterest or refusals.

In contrast, women's sexual initiations, and by extension women's perpetration of verbal sexual coercion, deviate from prescribed gender roles. According to traditional gendered sexual scripts, women who initiate sex are acting like men. Although sexual scripts are evolving, women who initiate sex, regardless of their partners' interests, are viewed differently from men who initiate sex. Some view women's sexual initiations negatively, as inappropriate violations of their feminine role as sexually conservative or sexual only for men's pleasure in a committed relationship. For example, Seal et al. (2007) described diverse negative reactions of men to women who assertively (but not coercively) asked for sex or made specific sexual requests (e.g., condom use). Others view women's sexual initiations more positively, precisely because they violate traditional scripts (Gavey, 2005); yet sexually assertive women are still at risk for being derogated as "sluts" or with other terms used to constrain female sexual behavior (Holland et al., 2004). As Gavey (2005) notes, without sociocultural discourses about (acceptable) female sexual agency, it is not always easy to differentiate between women's sexual initiations and women's sexually coercive behavior.

We suggest that comparisons of women's and men's verbally coercive sexual behaviors are necessarily asymmetric because these behaviors are interpreted in terms of gendered norms and sexual scripts. In fact, research substantiates this conclusion; observers view the same verbally coercive acts by hypothetical men and women in a heterosexual context as reflecting men's aggression but women's promiscuity (Oswald & Russell, 2006). This is not to say that women are incapable of coercing men into sex or that such behaviors are more acceptable. Rather, our point is that the meanings attached to women's sexual coercion of men meaningfully differ from the meanings attached to men's sexual coercion of women.

Gendered norms and scripts also are evident in research describing and explaining gender differences in verbal sexual coercion. For example, Motley (2008) asked undergraduate college students (heterosexuality presumed) about specific premises used to verbally coerce sex (i.e., "You should have sex with me because of . . ."). Coercive men typically expressed that women "owed" them sex (due to the length of the relationship, love for the partner, past sexual precedence, level of arousal), whereas coercive women typically expressed that men who refused sex were inadequate or gay. In other words, gendered expectations based on the have/hold and male sexual drive discourses were invoked to coerce women and men, respectively. In another study, Schatzel-Murphy, Harris, Knight, and Milburn (2009) suggest that women's sexual coercion of men (defined broadly, including seduction, manipulation, intoxication, or force) reflected women's unmet needs for interpersonal connection; in contrast, Schatzel-Murphy et al. suggest that the same behaviors enacted by men toward women reflected men's unmet needs for power and control. In these studies, research participants and researchers alike provided evidence for normative understandings of gender and heterosex; at the same time, research participants and researchers alike also used these discourses to make sense of verbal sexual coercion experiences.

Responses to Verbal Coercion

Gendered sexual scripts help explain the sexual coercion of women by men more readily than the coercion of men by women. Sex differences in response to unwanted sexual advances also converge with traditional scripts. For example, O'Sullivan et al. (1998) found that women reported a wider range of and stronger resistance to unwanted sexual advances than men, which the authors interpreted as meaning that unwanted sexual activity was more aversive and threatening to women.

Men who are verbally sexually coerced breach gendered sexual scripts prescribing male dominance. Men who refuse sex, even coercive pressure for sex, also violate expectations based on the male sexual drive discourse, making men vulnerable to capitulation. In addition, men who are verbally coerced by women may be denigrated due to expected gender differences in size and strength. In a heterosexual context, male victims of verbal coercion are seen as having greater control than women victims; in turn, greater victim control predicts greater responsibility (Katz, Moore, & Tkachuk, 2007). That is, a man who is verbally coerced by a woman is expected to extricate himself from the situation. Not surprisingly, men who experience coerced sex (perpetrated by either women or men) often are devalued as weak or unmasculine; alternatively, they are seen as choosing to be coerced into sex (Davies & Roger, 2006). Such conceptions of male victimization are problematic for many reasons, including the singular focus on the attributes and behaviors of the (male) victim rather than the (female) perpetrator.

Research describing gender differences in emotional responses to sexual coercion also cannot be interpreted without considering norms about gender and heterosex. In general, sexual violations of both women and men are routinely minimized by both observers and victims themselves (Anderson & Doherty, 2008). No studies to date have directly examined gender differences in responses to dating partner verbal sexual coercion. However, in the broader sexual literature (involving various forms of coercion and relationship contexts), boys and men are much more likely than girls or women to minimize their own coerced sexual experiences. For example, among high school students who experienced unwanted sexual activity (not necessarily verbal sexual coercion or by a dating partner), about half of the male students reported that it had no effect on them. In addition, female students were significantly more likely to report feeling dirty, scared, angry, cheap, or duped (Jackson, Cram, & Seymour, 2000). Similarly, O'Sullivan et al. (1998) found significant gender differences in the degree of upset reported by college students after sexual victimization by dating partners; more than 40% of men but only 6% of women reported no effect. As noted by Gavey (2005), it is possible to accept such responses at face value. It is also possible, however, that minimization allows boys and men to ignore the potential threat of such experiences to their sense of masculinity.

Verbal Sexual Coercion and Sexual Consent in Relational Context

As noted in the first section of this chapter, sexual consent is legally presumed once individuals reach a state-designated age of adulthood (McGregor, 2005). In addition, sexual consent in a relationship is often presumed as a function of one's past sexual experiences. More specifically, sexual consent at one point in time may imply future consent across partners, across time, and within a sequence of sexual activity. These presumptions of sexual consent increase the risk for verbal sexual coercion specifically in intimate relationships.

In many dating relationships, expectations about sexual intimacy may be shaped by knowledge of a partner's past sexual experiences. That is, sexually experienced adolescents are often expected, and thus pressured, to engage in sex when they begin new dating relationships. For example, in Hyde et al.'s (2008) study of high school students, some girls said that male partners pressured them into having sex because the girls had previously consented to sex with other boys. Similarly, Bay-Cheng and Eliseo-Arras (2008) described how one college student's new partner knew that she had previously performed oral sex on another man; the new partner used that knowledge to verbally pressure her into performing oral sex on him as well. The implication here is that there is no legitimate reason to refuse a new partner after one's first time.

Consensual sexual experiences within a specific dating relationship also may lead to presumptions of future consent, increasing the likelihood that verbal coercion will occur. In other words, after a person consents to sex with a partner at one point in time, she or he also is presumed to be consenting to future sex with that same partner. This sexual precedence explains why sexual refusal behaviors are viewed as less legitimate in couples with a history of consensual sex as compared to couples without such a history (Shotland & Goodstein, 1992). The presumption of consent can create both entitlement to exert coercive pressure and obligation to submit to such pressure. In some cases, perpetrators may exert pressure for reciprocity. For example, Bay-Cheng and Eliseo-Arras (2008) reported that a male partner verbally pressured his girlfriend to perform oral sex on him after he performed it on her. In other cases, perpetrators may invoke obligation and guilt based on an expectation for continued sexual access (e.g., Livingston et al., 2004). These expectations also were evident in Seal et al.'s (2007) study of men's narratives about sex in established relationships. Most men perceived that partners are obligated to make each other happy by engaging in sex even in the absence of desire. As such, most men felt that they had the right to demand sex and to expect compliance from their partners; pressure and persistence were common, as were threats to the relationship and demands for alternative activities (i.e., pressure for oral instead of vaginal penetration). Seal et al. concluded that men's perceived sexual entitlement was due to beliefs about access to their specific sexual partner based on sexual precedence, not on men's rights to have sex with women generally.

Perhaps the most controversial area involving sexual precedence and consent involves the typical heterosexual progression from less intimate (e.g., kissing, hugging) to more intimate (e.g., genital contact) levels of sexual activity, often culminating in (male) orgasm (Gavey, 2005). In a study of American college students, Hall (1998) found that most young couples proceed through sequences of sexual activity without consenting at each juncture. Sexual consent to certain sexual behaviors implied consent for other more intimate behaviors; consent was often given only once, and the sequence proceeded until expressed resistance was encountered. Such presumptions coupled with the tendency for sexual consent to be expressed indirectly via nonverbal channels (Hickman & Muehlenhard, 1999) help explain why verbal sexual coercion is often attributed to miscommunication (Abbey et al., 2004).

Nevertheless, attributing verbal sexual coercion to miscommunication is both incomplete and problematic. First, miscommunication exonerates the coercive partner for not seeking clear or genuine affirmation or consent. Second, miscommunication obscures the fact that typical sexual progressions described by Hall (1998) privilege sexual pursuit over sexual reticence. Third, miscommunication mistakenly connotes the idea that sexual negotiations are gender-neutral, overlooking typical gender differences in preferences for sexual consent. Among American college students, for example, women are more likely than men to indicate that consent should be given before sexual activity ("assume no until you hear yes"), whereas men are more likely than women to assume consent until they hear otherwise ("assume yes until you hear no"). In addition, women are more likely than men to believe that relationship commitment does not nullify the need to ensure consent and that consent is a process rather than a one-time event (Humphreys & Herold, 2007). In short, presumptions of consent within dating couples privilege the pursuer at the expense of the pursued. When sexual pursuits become verbally coercive, miscommunication provides a useful, albeit inaccurate, cover story to neutralize the event.

CONCLUSION

Although verbally coercive dating partners do not physically force others into sex, coercive partners exert overwhelming or unrelenting psychological pressure. Ultimately victims capitulate to escape partner pressure and to avoid the negative consequences of persistent sexual refusal (Livingston et al., 2004). Heterosexual victims of verbal sexual coercion are perceived to have more control than victims of rape, which explains the greater responsibility attributed to verbal sexual coercion victims, especially men (Katz et al., 2007). Verbal coercion due to psychological pressure also may be minimized as harmless and inconsequential. We conclude by briefly challenging these victim-blaming attitudes about control and responsibility.

Verbal sexual coercion cannot be controlled by victims whose sexual refusals are ignored. Although direct refusals may curtail coercion in some situations (e.g., Testa & Derman, 1999), sexual pursuit commonly continues even after an initiator is told "no" unequivocally (e.g., Struckman-Johnson, Struckman-Johnson, & Anderson, 2003). In addition, surrender may allow individuals to avoid escalation to increasingly forceful tactics. In particular, men's verbal coercion of young women tends to co-occur with psychologically abusive behaviors, including insults (Starratt et al., 2008), controlling behaviors (Goetz & Shackelford, 2009; Katz & Myhr, 2008), or even physically violent behaviors (Katz et al., 2002; Katz, Moore, & May, 2008; White & Smith, 2009). In some cases surrender may feel and be safer than resistance.

The tactics of verbal sexual coercion also should not be trivialized; psychological pressure can be just as or even more threatening than physical force. Consider the potential long-term effects of having one's reputation ruined ("I'll tell everyone that you're a fag/slut") as a consequence of refusing sexual advances. Doesn't every person have the right to refuse sex without fear of social ruin? Sexually coercive psychological pressure is not necessarily harmless; such accusations and derogations "enter the social world with effect" (Gavey, 2005, p. 105).

The idea that psychological pressure by a verbally coercive partner can be overcome (controlled) by sufficient victim resistance sidesteps the idea of shared responsibility for sex in relationships. Shouldn't sexually coercive persons heed their partner's lack of enthusiastic (or even unequivocal) consent? Focusing on presumably controllable resistance to presumably trivial psychological pressure disproportionately shifts attention to victims of verbally coerced sex. Such a focus is unwarranted without corresponding attention to perpetrators. Furthermore, neither victim nor perpetrator behaviors can be fully understood without considering the larger gendered and relational contexts of heterosexual intimacy. In turn, contextualized understandings of how and why verbal coercion occurs are needed to effectively combat verbal sexual coercion in heterosexual dating relationships.

REFERENCES

Abbey, A., BeShears, R., Clinton-Sherrod, A. M., & McAuslan, P. (2004). Similarities and differences in women's sexual assault experiences based on tactics used by the perpetrator. *Psychology of Women Quarterly, 28,* 323–332.

Anderson, I., & Doherty, K. (2008). *Accounting for rape: Psychology, feminism, and discourse analysis in the study of sexual violence.* New York: Routledge.

Bay-Cheng, L. Y., & Eliseo-Arras, R. K. (2008). The making of unwanted sex: Gendered and neoliberal norms in college women's unwanted sexual experiences. *Journal of Sex Research, 45,* 386–397.

Beres, M. A. (2007). 'Spontaneous' sexual consent: An analysis of sexual consent literature. *Feminism & Psychology, 17,* 93–108.

Bourke, J. (2007). *Rape: Sex, violence, history.* New York: Virago.

Brownridge, D. (2006). Intergenerational transmission and dating violence victimization: Evidence from a sample of female university students in Manitoba. *Canadian Journal of Community Mental Health, 25,* 75–93.

Byers, E. S. (1996). How well does the traditional sexual script explain sexual coercion? Review of a program of research. *Journal of Psychology and Human Sexuality, 8,* 7–25.

Craig, M. E. (1990). Coercive sexuality in dating relationships: A situational model. *Clinical Psychology Review, 10,* 395–423.

Crown, L., & Roberts, L. J. (2007). Against their will: Young women's nonagentic sexual experiences. *Journal of Social and Personal Relationships, 24,* 385–405.

Davies, M., & Rogers, P. (2006). Perceptions of male victims in depicted sexual assaults: A review of the literature. *Aggression and Violent Behavior, 11,* 367–377.

DeGue, S., & DeLillo, S. (2004). Understanding perpetrators of nonphysical sexual coercion: Characteristics of those who cross the line. *Violence and Victims, 19,* 673–688.

Doroszewicz, K., & Forbes, G. B. (2008). Experiences with dating aggression and sexual coercion among Polish college students. *Journal of Interpersonal Violence, 23,* 58–73.

Finkelhor, D., & Yllo, K. (1987). *License to rape: Sexual abuse of wives.* New York: Free Press.

Gavey, N. (2005). *Just sex? The cultural scaffolding of rape.* New York: Routledge.

Goetz, A. T., & Shackelford, T. K. (2009). Sexual coercion in intimate relationships: A comparative analysis of the effects of women's infidelity and men's dominance and control. *Archives of Sexual Behavior, 38,* 226–234.

Gowen, L. K., Feldman, S. S., Diaz, R., & Yisrael, D. S. (2004). A comparison of the sexual behaviors and attitudes of adolescent girls with older vs. similar-aged boyfriends. *Journal of Youth and Adolescence, 33,* 167–175.

Hall, D. E. (1998). Consent for sexual behavior in a college student population. Electronic *Journal of Human Sexuality, 1,* http://www.ejhs.org/volume1/consent1.htm.

Harned, M. S. (2001). Abused women or abused men? An examination of the context and outcomes of dating violence. *Violence and Victims, 16,* 269–285.

Hickman, S. E., & Muehlenhard, C. L. (1999). By the semi-mystical appearance of a condom: How young women and men communicate sexual consent in heterosexual situations. *Journal of Sex Research, 36,* 258–272.

Hines, D. A. (2007). Predictors of sexual coercion against women and men: A multilevel, multinational study of university students. *Archives of Sexual Behavior, 36,* 403–422.

Hines, D. A., & Saudino, K. J. (2003). Gender differences in psychological, physical, and sexual aggression among college students using the Revised Conflict Tactics Scales. *Violence and Victims, 18,* 197–217.

Holland, J., Ramazanoglu, C., Sharpe, S., & Thompson, R. (2004). *The male in the head: Young people, heterosexuality, and power.* London: Tufnell.

Holloway, W. (1984). Women's power in heterosexual sex. *Women's Studies International Forum, 7,* 63–68.

Humphreys, T., & Herold, E. (2007). Sexual consent in heterosexual relationships: Development of a new measure. *Sex Roles, 57,* 305–315.

Hyde, A., Drennan, J., Howlett, E., & Brady, D. (2008). Heterosexual experiences of secondary school pupils in Ireland: Sexual coercion in context. *Culture, Health & Sexuality, 10,* 479–493.

Jackson, S., Cram F., & Seymour, F. W. (2000). Violence and sexual coercion in high school students' dating relationships. *Journal of Family Violence, 15,* 23–36.

Kaestle, C. E. (2009). Sexual insistence and disliked sexual activities in young adulthood: Differences by gender and relationship characteristics. *Perspectives on Sexual and Reproductive Health, 41,* 33–39.

Katz, J., Carino, A., & Hilton, A. (2002). Perceived verbal conflict behaviors associated with physical aggression and sexual coercion in dating relationships: A gender-sensitive analysis. *Violence and Victims, 17,* 93–109.

Katz, J., Kuffel S. W., & Brown, F. A. (2006). Leaving a sexually coercive dating partner: A prospective test of the investment model. *Psychology of Women Quarterly, 30,* 267–275.

Katz, J., Moore, J. A., & May, P. (2008). Physical and sexual covictimization from dating partners: A distinct type of interpersonal abuse? *Violence Against Women, 14,* 961–980.

Katz, J., Moore, J. A., & Tkachuk, S. (2007). Verbal sexual coercion and perceived victim responsibility: Mediating effects of perceived control. *Sex Roles, 57,* 235–247.

Katz, J., & Myhr, L. (2008). Perceived conflict patterns and relationship quality associated with verbal sexual coercion by male dating partners. *Journal of Interpersonal Violence, 23,* 798–814.

Koss, M. P., & Oros, C. J. (1982). Sexual Experiences Survey: A research instrument investigating sexual aggression and victimization. *Journal of Consulting and Clinical Psychology, 50,* 455–457.

Littleton, H. L., & Axsom, D. (2003). Rape and seduction scripts of university students: Implications for rape attributions and unacknowledged rape. *Sex Roles, 49,* 465–475.

Livingston, J. A., Buddie, A. M., Testa, M., & VanZile-Tamsen, C. (2004). The role of sexual precedence in verbal sexual coercion. *Psychology of Women Quarterly, 28,* 287–297.

Lyndon, A. E., White, J. W., & Kadlec, K. M. (2007). Manipulation and force as sexual coercion tactics: Conceptual and empirical differences. *Aggressive Behavior, 33,* 291–303.

McGregor, J. (2005). *Is it rape? On acquaintance rape and taking women's consent seriously.* New York: Ashgate.

Motley, M. T. (2008). Verbal coercion to unwanted sexual intimacy: How coercion messages operate. In M. T. Motley (Ed.), *Studies in applied interpersonal communication* (pp. 185–203). Thousand Oaks, CA: Sage.

Muehlenhard, C. L., & Peterson, Z. D. (2004). Conceptualizing sexual violence: Socially acceptable coercion and other controversies. In A. G. Miller (Ed.), *The social psychology of good and evil* (pp. 240–268). New York: Guilford.

Offman, A. & Matheson, K. (2004). The sexual self-perceptions of young women experiencing abuse in dating relationships. *Sex Roles, 51,* 551–559.

O'Leary, K. D., & Williams, M. C. (2006). Agreement about acts of aggression in marriage. *Journal of Family Psychology, 20,* 656–662.

O'Sullivan, L. F., Byers, E. S., & Finkelman, L. (1998). A comparison of male and female college students' experiences of sexual coercion. *Psychology of Women Quarterly, 22,* 177–195.

Oswald, D. L., & Russell, D. L. (2006). Perceptions of sexual coercion in heterosexual dating relationships: The role of aggressor gender and tactics. *Journal of Sex Research, 43,* 87–95.

Patton, W., & Mannison, M. (1995). Sexual coercion in dating situations among university students: Preliminary Australian data. *Australian Journal of Psychology, 47,* 66–72.

Poitras, M., & Lavoie, F. (1995). A study of the prevalence of sexual coercion in adolescent heterosexual dating relationships in a Quebec sample. *Violence and Victims, 10,* 299–312.

Schatzel-Murphy, E., Harris, D. A., Knight, R. A., & Milburn, M. A. (2009). Sexual coercion in men and women: Similar behaviors, different predictors. *Archives of Sexual Behavior, 38,* 974–986.

Schulhofer, S. J. (1998). *Unwanted sex: The culture of intimidation and the failure of law*. Cambridge: Harvard University Press.

Seal, D. W., & Ehrhardt, A. A. (2003). Masculinity and urban men: Perceived scripts for courtship, romantic, and sexual interactions with women. *Culture, Health, and Sexuality, 5*, 295–319.

Seal, D. W., O'Sullivan, L. F., & Ehrhardt, A. A. (2007). Miscommunications and misinterpretations: Men's scripts about sexual communication and unwanted sex in interactions with women. In M. Kimmel (Ed.), *The sexual self: The construction of sexual scripts* (pp. 141–161). Nashville, TN: Vanderbilt University Press.

Shackelford, T. K., & Goetz, A. T. (2004). Men's sexual coercion in intimate relationships: Development and initial validation of the sexual coercion in intimate relationships scale. *Violence and Victims, 19*, 541–556.

Shotland, R. L., & Goodstein, L. (1992). Sexual precedence reduces the perceived legitimacy of sexual arousal: An examination of attributions concerning date rape and consensual sex. *Personality and Social Psychology Bulletin, 18*, 756–764.

Slashinski, M. J., Coker, A. J., & Davis, K. E. (2003). Physical aggression, forced sex, and stalking victimization by a dating partner: An analysis of the National Violence Against Women Survey. *Violence and Victims, 18*, 595–617.

Starratt, V. G., Goetz, A. T., Shackelford, T. K., McKibbin, W. F., & Stewart-Williams, S. (2008). Men's partner-directed insults and sexual coercion in intimate relationships. *Journal of Family Violence, 23*, 315–323.

Straus, M. A., Hamby, S. L., Boney-McCoy, S., & Sugarman, D. B. (1996). The Revised Conflict Tactics Scales (CTS2): Development and preliminary psychometric data. *Journal of Family Issues, 17*, 283–316.

Struckman-Johnson, C. (1988). Forced sex on dates: It happens to men, too. *Journal of Sex Research, 24*, 234–241.

Struckman-Johnson, C., Struckman-Johnson, D., & Anderson, P. B. (2003). Tactics of sexual coercion: When men and women won't take no for an answer. *Journal of Sex Research, 40*, 76–86.

Testa, M., & Derman, K. H. (1999). The differential correlates of sexual coercion and rape. *Journal of Interpersonal Violence, 14*, 548–561.

Testa, M., VanZile-Tamsen, C., Livingston, J. A., & Koss, M. P. (2004). Assessing women's experiences of sexual aggression using the Sexual Experiences Survey: Evidence for validity and implications for research. *Psychology of Women Quarterly, 28*, 256–265.

Tyler, K. A., & Johnson, K. A. (2006). Trading sex: Voluntary or coerced? The experiences of homeless youth. *Journal of Sex Research, 43*, 208–216.

VanderLaan, D. P., & Vasey, P. L. (2009). Patterns of sexual coercion in heterosexual and non-heterosexual men and women. *Archives of Sexual Behavior, 38*, 987–999.

Vogel, R. E., & Himelein, M. J. (1995). Dating and sexual victimization: An analysis of risk factors among precollege women. *Journal of Criminal Justice, 23*, 153–162.

Waldner-Haugrud, L. K., & Magruder, B. (1995). Male and female sexual victimization in dating relationships: Gender differences in coercion techniques and outcomes. *Violence and Victims, 10*, 203–215.

White, J. W., & Smith, P. H. (2009). Covariation in the use of physical and sexual intimate partner aggression among adolescent and college-age men: A longitudinal analysis. *Violence Against Women, 15*, 24–43.

Chapter 5

Intimate Partner Violence as Workplace Violence

Impact on Women's Mental Health and Work Performance

Michele A. Paludi

INTRODUCTION

In January 2011, media attention was once again focused on intimate partner violence and the workplace. That month Prudential Financial, Inc., joined the Corporate Alliance to End Partner Violence. This organization, the sole national organization of its kind founded by business leaders, deals with preventing intimate partner violence from impacting the workplace. This alliance provides research, training, policy, and program development and crisis consultation for member organizations. Prudential joined other corporate members of the alliance—including Mary Kay, Inc.; Rutgers University; State Farm Insurance; the Wireless Foundation; Eastman Kodak; Enterprise Rent-A-Car; Lifetime Television; Liz Claiborne, Inc.; and the World Bank Group—dedicated to preventing intimate partner violence from entering the workplace and educating employees about this form of violence.

The need for this alliance is supported by the startling personal accounts as well as statistics. For example:

Barbara Cavalier had been married to her husband, Chris Cavalier, for seven years. During the course of their marriage, Chris had been abusive toward Barbara. When he put a gun to her head, she decided to leave him. For six months her living arrangements were kept secret. One day Chris walked into the Elmwood siding supply business and saw Barbara where she was working as a data entry clerk. Subsequently Chris walked into the store armed with two guns, a .45-caliber automatic pistol and a .357-caliber Magnum revolver. Chris killed Barbara and her coworker Stephanie Revolta, who had tried to defuse the situation. Stephanie had placed a 911 call, but by the time assistance arrived, Barbara and Stephanie were dead. Chris also took his own life. Barbara's coworkers reported that Chris had been harassing Barbara all day, calling her at work and stealing her truck. Authorities had found a note in Chris's house in which he assigned power of attorney and listed valuables that he wanted to give away. This behavior led police to believe that Chris had planned the murders that day (Paludi, Nydegger & Paludi, 2006).

Ellen works for a small shipping company in the western Canadian city of Vancouver. She has been unhappily married to Paul for more than 20 years, and she and her two daughters bear the brunt of Paul's verbal taunts and controlling behavior. Although he has never physically abused the children, he often beats Ellen so severely that vicious bruises cover her arms and legs, and she regularly lies to her coworkers about their origin, claiming clumsiness, embarrassed by their true cause. At least once a month Ellen is so badly hurt that she must stay out of work. In the past two years alone she has lost 22 days of work and thousands of dollars in wages.

One night, Paul angrily smacks Ellen's younger daughter, and she falls down the stairs, cutting open her knee. After years of abuse Ellen has finally had enough and leaves. She moves in with a friend and changes her phone number and personal email address. For a while things are fine. But soon Ellen begins receiving threatening prank phone calls at the office and nasty emails to her work email account. She thinks that it might be Paul, and her suspicions are confirmed when one evening she discovers him waiting for her in the office parking lot. In a dark and menacing tone Paul threatens to kill her and their children unless she returns to him.

She doesn't know who to turn to or where to go. For years she has been hiding her abuse from her friends, family, coworkers, and employers, and the threats continue to escalate (Soroptimist International of the Americas, 2007).

The Occupational Safety and Health Administration (2010) reported that approximately 2 million employees like Barbara and Ellen are victims of workplace violence each year. Homicide is the leading cause of occupational death for women in the United States and is the second-leading cause of occupational death for men (Knefel & Bryant, 2004; Lieber, 2011; National Institute for Occupational Safety and Health, 2010; Paludi, Wilmot & Speach, 2010; Reeves & O'Leary-Kelly, 2007; Swanberg & Logan, 2007). The National Institute for Occupational Health and Safety (2010) reported that women are 39% more likely than men to be victims of workplace violence.

In this chapter I review the incidence of intimate partner violence as a workplace concern and the empirical research on the impact of intimate partner violence on women's emotional and physical health, self-concept, interpersonal relationships with coworkers and supervisors, and career goals. Recommendations are offered for employers in exercising reasonable care in responding to women employees who are victims of intimate partner violence, including developing and enforcing effective policy and investigatory procedures and training programs on intimate partner violence awareness.

INCIDENCE OF INTIMATE PARTNER VIOLENCE AT THE WORKPLACE

Intimate partner violence includes intense criticisms and put-downs, verbal harassment, sexual coercion and assault, pushing, shoving, physical attacks, choking, stalking, denial of access to resources, and murder (Paludi, Wilmot, & Speach, 2010). According to the Occupational Safety and Health Administration (2010, p. 1), workplace violence "can occur at or outside the workplace and can range from threats and verbal abuse to physical assaults and homicide." Knefel and Bryant (2004, p. 582) define workplace violence as "any actual or attempted act of force-physical, verbal and sexual-against person(s) and/or organization(s) that cause injury to intended and/or unintended target(s) occurring within and due to the occupational context."

Men who are likely to be victims of workplace violence are employees who exchange money with the public; deliver goods, passengers, and services; work alone or in small groups; and have extensive contact with the public (e.g., drive taxis or work in retail or hospital settings) (Paludi, Nydegger, & Paludi, 2006; Probst, Estrada, & Brown, 2008; Worthington, 2000). Research indicates that victims are those on the front line (Kelloway, Barling, & Harrell, 2006; Paludi, Nydegger, & Paludi, 2006; Schaffer, Casteel, & Kraus, 2002). For women, although they may be at risk because they are employed in these same jobs, more of them experience workplace violence from current or former mates or spouses (i.e., intimates). Approximately 26 million women are victims of intimate partner violence each year (Swanberg & Logan, 2005).

Straus, Gelles, and Steinmetz (1980) reported that one out of every six couples engage in at least one violent act each year. Thus, over the course of a relationship approximately one-fourth of couples will experience intimate partner violence. Women victims of intimate partner violence account for one-fourth of all women who are murdered in a given year (McHugh & Frieze, 2006; Rathus & Feindler, 2004). More women in the United States are victimized by their spouses/mates than are harmed because of reported automobile accidents, muggings, and rapes combined (Swanberg, Logan, & Macke, 2005). Tjaden and Thoennes (2000) reported that over a lifetime, the prevalence of intimate partner violence for women is triple the prevalence for men.

These statistics include intimate partner violence across all races and ethnic groups; among women in urban, rural, and suburban areas; and in lesbian, gay, and heterosexual relationships (Coleman, 1991; McHugh & Frieze, 2006; Paludi, Nydegger, & Paludi, 2006; Potocziak, Murot, Crosbie-Burnett, & Potoczni, 2003). While women are more likely to be victims of intimate partner violence, men may be battered (Horne, 1999; McHugh & Frieze, 2006). Men batter because they want control in the relationship. Women, however, batter in self-defense because of fear of being murdered (Babcock, Miller, & Siard, 2003). Horne (1999) found that more women are seriously injured or killed by male partners each year than are men by female partners.

In addition, research suggested that the incidence of same-sex intimate partner violence is similar to that of heterosexual intimate partner violence (McHugh & Frieze, 2006; Potocziak et al. 2003). Furthermore, the Fourth United Nations International Conference on Women concluded that "in all societies . . . women and girls are subjected to physical, sexual and psychological abuse that cuts across lines of income, class and culture" (Walker, 1999, p. 21). Tran & DesJardins (2000) reported that the incidence of intimate partner violence experienced by Vietnamese and Korean communities is similar to the incidence rates in the United States. In addition, Horne (1999) noted that intimate partner violence in Russia is four to five times more frequent than in the United States.

IMPACT OF INTIMATE PARTNER VIOLENCE ON ORGANIZATIONS

Research conducted by the Corporate Alliance to End Partner Violence, Liz Claiborne, and Safe Horizon (Corporate Alliance to End Partner Violence, 2007) reported that while chief executive officers believe that only 6% of their full-time employees are victims of intimate partner violence, more than 26% of women in the workplace admit to being victimized by a mate or spouse. In addition, 24% of employees report knowing a coworker who is a victim of intimate partner violence. The Corporate Alliance to End Partner Violence (2005) reported that 21% of full-time employed adults were victims of intimate partner violence; 64% indicated that their work performance had been impacted significantly by the violence. According to the Centers for Disease Control and Prevention (2008), victims of intimate partner violence lose approximately 8 million days of work annually. This translates into approximately 32,000 full-time jobs. In addition, the cost of intimate partner violence to the U.S. economy is more than $8.3 billion, including medical care, mental health care, and lost productivity from work.

For workplaces in the United States, intimate partner violence costs $727.8 million in lost productivity annually. Furthermore, direct medical and mental health care services cost employers approximately $6 billion each year. Willman's (2007) review of Fortune 1000 companies indicated that 49% of these corporate leaders reported that intimate partner violence had harmful effects on the productivity of their organizations. In addition, 47% indicated that the violence had a harmful impact on attendance. Furthermore, 44% indicated that the violence was harmful to their health care costs, thereby impacting the organization's bottom line. The average absenteeism rate of victims of intimate partner violence is approximately 30% higher than the average employee absenteeism rate (American Institute on Domestic Violence, 2009).

IMPACT OF INTIMATE PARTNER VIOLENCE ON VICTIMS

Swanberg and Logan (2007) suggested that the impact of intimate partner violence on women employees contributed to women's inability to concentrate and solve problems at work, perform their job, go to work, remain at work, and keep their jobs. Prework interference prevented 56% of women in their study from going to work as a consequence of physical restraint, having their clothes cut up, being beaten, or being denied access to their car. Wetterstein et al. (2004) found that battered women experience prework incidents of violence at least once a week.

Interference with women's employment at the workplace included the following behaviors: phone harassment, harassment of the women's supervisors, threatening comments, stalking, and being physically forced to leave work. Women participants in research by Swanberg and Logan (2005) offered examples of ways that intimate partner violence impacted their work. For example:

- I was working at a restaurant and he showed up outside and just started beating on the back door. We had closed up and we were cleaning up for inspection and stuff and the manager come and told me that he was out there. I of course went outside. I could see that he was drunk and he was very angry.... He saw me talking with someone.... He started throwing me around the parking lot and they called the law and I got fired.
- I was the food stamp caseworker; it was the best money I ever made. He would pop up from nowhere, if I was gone too long [from my chair] he'd know it and then the phone calls would start from the outside phone booth. I had no idea how he knew my every move. If I stayed too late at work, the phone calls would start from home. The unpredictability was most stressful.... I was afraid I'd lose my job.

In Swanberg and Logan's (2005) research, although 46% of women informed their managers about the intimate partner violence that they were experiencing,

54% chose to remain silent. Furthermore, 43% of the women informed one of their coworkers about the battering; 57% did not. Women who do not disclose the battering remain silent at work for several reasons, including fear of losing their job, being ashamed of being battered, being ashamed of their appearance (e.g., bruises, broken bones), and being frightened.

For batterers, the workplace provides a site where they know their victims' whereabouts throughout the day. Thus, the workplace is not a safe haven for women victims of intimate partner violence; the violence spills over into the workplace. Furthermore, Ridley (2004) reported that 74% of batterers indicated that they had easy access to their partner's workplace. In addition, 21% of these men had contacted their partner at the company in violation of a restraining order, and 48% indicated that they could not concentrate at their own job because of their preoccupation with their partner. Of these men, Ridley reported 19% having a workplace accident and 42% being late for work because of battering their mate.

Swanberg, Macke, and Logan (2006, p. 573) also noted that "When partner violence traverses the boundaries of women's jobs, the victimized partner is no longer the only victim. Other people on the workplace premises, including supervisors, other workers, and customers, are at risk for injury or some other form of trauma."

The American Bar Association Commission on Domestic Violence (1999, p. 16) noted the following observable behaviors that suggest intimate partner violence and can assist employers in prevention. This listing may be provided to managers during training:

a. Unexplained tardiness and absences
b. Unplanned use of leave time
c. Lack of concentration
d. A tendency to remain isolated from coworkers or a reluctance to participate in social events
e. Discomfort when communicating with others
f. Disruptive phone calls or email
g. Frequent financial problems indicating lack of access to money
h. Unexplained bruises or injuries
i. Noticeable change in use of makeup (to cover up injuries)
j. Inappropriate clothes (e.g., sunglasses worn inside the building, turtleneck worn in the summer)
k. Sudden changes of address or reluctance to divulge where she is staying
l. Court appearances

Research on intimate partner violence has documented impact on several areas of functioning, including emotional/psychological, physiological or health related, career, interpersonal, and self-perception (Lundberg-Love & Marmion, 2006; McHugh, Livingston, & Frieze, 2008; O'Leary & Maiuro, 2001; Reeves & O'Leary, 2007; Swanberg et al., 2006). The following are reported physical/

health-related effects of intimate partner violence: headaches, tiredness, respiratory problems, substance abuse, sleep disturbances, eating disorders, lethargy, gastrointestinal disorders, post-traumatic stress disorder (PTSD), the hostage syndrome, and inability to concentrate (Lundberg-Love & Wilkerson, 2006; McHugh & Frieze, 2006; Walker, 2006; Zorza, 2002).

In addition, battered women experience injuries including bruises, cuts, concussions, black eyes, broken bones, scars from burns, knife wounds, loss of hearing and/or vision, and joint damage (Feblinger, 2008; Lundberg-Love & Wilkerson, 2006). Pregnant women who experience intimate partner violence face the risk of severe outcomes for their fetus as well as themselves (Sagrestano, Carroll, Rodriguez, & Nuwayhid, 2004). The impact of intimate partner violence on social and interpersonal relationships includes the following: withdrawal, fear of new people, lack of trust, and changes in social network patterns at work (Lundberg-Love & Wilkerson, 2006; Swanberg et al., 2006).

Examples of emotional/psychological effects of intimate partner violence include, but are not limited to, guilt, denial, withdrawal from social settings, shame, depression, fear, anger, anxiety, phobias, isolation, fear of crime, helplessness, frustration, shock, and decreased self-esteem (Cunradi, Ames, & Moore, 2008; Swanberg et al., 2006).

Furthermore, these responses to intimate partner violence as a workplace concern are not independent of each other. Women victims of intimate partner violence may receive threatening emails, calls, and/or faxes at work. This has implications for women employees' mental state and contributes to their inability to concentrate and their failure to follow their job responsibilities and thus to being fired.

Lloyd and Taluc (1999) also reported that out of the 824 women in their sample, 18% indicated that they had experienced intimate partner violence, 11.9% had incurred more severe violence at the hand of their mate or spouse, and 40.3% said that they had been coerced and threatened by their mate or spouse. In addition, 28.4% had experienced abuse at the criminal assault level. These women reported experiencing unemployment, emotional and physical health problems, and higher welfare rates than women who did not experience intimate partner violence.

Intimate partner violence also has direct implications for a mother's emotional well-being in regard to effective parenting. The dysfunction and disorganization of the home offer little or no support, structure, nurturance, or supervision for children (Walker, 1999). Children are often neglected by mothers who are too emotionally and physically abused to care for them (Black & Newman, 2000). Walker (1999) and Graham and Rawlings (1999) estimated that each year approximately 3.3 million children in the United States between the ages of 3 and 17 years are at risk of exposure to their mothers being battered by a male spouse or mate.

Most battered women remain in the violent relationship because they believe that their situation is inescapable. They feel helpless about changing their lives and fear that any action they take will contribute to additional violence, a fear that is justified (Butts Stahly, 1999; Zorza, 2002). Furthermore, cultural factors contribute to remaining silent to protect the family's honor (Marmion & Faulkner, 2006).

Battered women remain in violent relationships for several well-founded reasons (McHugh & Frieze, 2006; Paludi, 2002; Butts Stahly, 1996), including threats to her life and the lives of her children if she leaves the home, fear of not getting custody of her children, financial dependence, feelings of responsibility for keeping the relationship together, love for the batterer, and the batterer is not always violent.

Grothues & Marmion (2006) noted that women victims of intimate partner violence frequently attempt to leave the relationship; their attempts are thwarted by their partners, who exercise more control and coercion with threats. Furthermore, Grothues and Marmion (2006, p. 11) reported that economic issues must be taken into consideration when understanding women remaining in a violent relationship:

> Women who leave their spouse often have no good alternatives for housing or support for themselves or their children. Because of the nature of the abuse, which often involves increasing isolation from others, victims tend to have a very small support system.

Shelters are not readily available in all communities, and even this option has limitations and has an impact on the children. It is not simply a case of not wanting to leave; most women do wish to do so. However, the costs of leaving are significant.

We note that Butts Stahly's (1999) review of the National Crime Survey of the Department of Justice indicated that 70% of intimate partner violence occurs after the relationship has ended. Similar findings were reported by Birns (1999), who reported that women are at an increased risk for homicide following the breakup of a relationship, more so than women who remain in the relationship.

WORKPLACE RESPONSES

> We challenge the culture of violence when we ourselves act in the certainty that violence is no longer acceptable, that it's tired and outdated no matter how many cling to it in the stubborn belief that it still works and that it's still valid.
>
> Gerard Vanderhaar

Unlike other forms of workplace harassment (e.g., sexual, national origin, age, disability, and race harassment), there are no specific laws regarding workplace violence (Paludi, Paludi, & DeSouza, 2010). The Occupational Safety and Health Administration (2010) has maintained that intimate partner violence as a workplace concern (as well as workplace violence in general) should follow the General Duty Clause, which is Section 5 (a)(1) of the Occupational Safety Act. This clause requires employers in the United States to "furnish to each of his employees employment and a place of employment which are free from recognized hazards that are causing or are likely to cause death or serious physical harm to his employees." In addition, Section 5 (a)(2) of this act requires employers to "comply with occupational safety and health standards promulgated under this Act."

Prevention of intimate violence as a workplace concern includes policies, procedures, and training programs (Paludi, Wilmot, & Speach, 2010; Nydegger, Paludi, DeSouza, & Paludi, 2006). Organizations should have in place a zero-tolerance policy for intimate partner violence. Effective policies and procedures encourage employees to disclose their victimization to the organization (Paludi, Wilmot, & Speach, 2010). Components of effective policy statements and procedures and sample policies are provided in Paludi, Nydegger, and Paludi (2006) and Paludi, Wilmot, and Speach (2010).

Training programs for managers and supervisors on intimate partner violence include reasons why victims fear disclosing their abuse, skills in behaving compassionately and supportively to employees who disclose intimate partner violence, basic emergency procedures, and myths versus realities about intimate partner violence (Paludi & Paludi, 2000; Paludi, Wilmot, & Speach, 2010).

Swanberg et al. (2006) suggested that women who chose not to disclose the intimate partner violence to their employer did so because of stigma associated with the violence (e.g., embarrassment, shame, fear of being judged), safety-related concerns (e.g., threatened by the abuser not to tell anyone about the violence, didn't want coworkers to become involved), and concerns related to the work environment (e.g., didn't know anyone to tell about the violence, couldn't trust coworkers and supervisors with the disclosure, the abuser also worked for the same organization). These responses should be made part of the training for managers so they can understand reasons for silence and reasons why the employer must be supportive to victims of intimate partner violence.

Furthermore, Swanberg et al. (2006) reported that women victims of intimate partner violence who disclosed the abuse at work fared better in terms of having longer job tenure, low job-quitting rates, and higher wages. It is therefore recommended to include in a training program that disclosing the intimate partner violence at work does not translate into employees losing their jobs.

Corporate Alliance to End Partner Violence, Liz Claiborne, and Safe Horizon (Corporate Alliance to End Partner Violence, 2007) reported that 90% of employees believe that managers and supervisors should be trained in recognizing the warning signs of intimate partner violence. Training programs in intimate partner violence assist employees in feeling more confident in their ability to deal with dangerous situations and in their employer's ability to prevent and deal with violence. As Swanberg et al. (2006, p. 574) noted, "Educating employees about partner violence could help to demystify the disgrace associated with this social problem and consequently help reduce or eliminate the risk of partner violence entering into the workplace."

Several engineering solutions have been recommended for organizations in their preventative and reactive management programs on workplace violence (Middelkoop, Gilhooley, Ruepp, Polikoski, & Paludi, 2008; Paludi, Nydegger, & Paludi, 2006; Stewart & Kleiner, 1997). Engineering solutions involve modifying the workplace environment to make it safer for employees. Employer engineering solutions regarding intimate partner violence include (Paludi, Wilmot, & Speach, 2010):

a. Implementing a personalized safety plan.
b. Identifying the workplace in a restraining order for the victim.
c. Saving threatening email and voice messages.
d. Identifying parking arrangements; having security escort employees to their car.
e. Removing employees' name and phone number from an automated phone directory.
f. Rotating the employee's work site or assignment.
g. Posting phone numbers at work sites, including for employee assistance programs (EAPs), the security department, the National Domestic Violence Hotline, local domestic violence resources, and information on obtaining orders of protection.

Examples of personalized safety plans can be found in Paludi, Nydegger, and Paludi (2006).

Furthermore, victims of intimate partner violence must not be retaliated against in terms of human resource functions (Lemon, 2001; Randel & Wells, 2003). For example, employee victims should not be identified as tardy or absent if they have to go to counseling, court, or appointments with physicians and therapists. Performance appraisals should not penalize employee victims in regard to time management or absenteeism. While managers may not fully be aware of the employees' situation, the organization's human resources department must ensure protection for employee victims.

Employers should also offer family and medical leave to employee victims. Examples of family-friendly policies for victims of intimate partner violence include flexible work hours, on-site health services, time off/career break, and workplace relocation that provide employees with the opportunity to continue working for their employer at a safer and anonymous job site (Paludi, Vaccariello, Graham, Smith, Allen-Dicker, Kasprzak, & White, 2006; Swanberg et al., 2006). Examples of such policies are found in Paludi and Paludi (2006).

In addition, educational materials may be developed for distribution and posting throughout the workplace, including posters with tear-off tabs containing hotline phone numbers for domestic violence shelters.

Since an intimate batterer may be a coworker of the employee victim, it is recommended that employers consider adopting a consensual relationship policy (Paludi, Nydegger, & Paludi, 2006). Consensual relationships are not illegal, but they do cause difficulties for organizations for various reasons:

a. The situation involves one person exerting power over another.
b. The seduction of a much younger individual is usually involved.
c. Conflict of interest issues arise. For example, how can a supervisor fairly evaluate an employee with whom she or he is having a sexual relationship?

d. The potential for exploitation and abuse is high.
   e. The potential for retaliatory harassment is high when the sexual relationship ceases.
   f. Other individuals may be affected and may make accusations of favoritism (Paludi, Nydegger, & Paludi, 2006, pp. 79–80).

Sample consensual relationship policies can be found in Paludi and Barickman (1998).

Women who have left a battering relationship report that they learned about intimate partner violence from listening to an EAP counselor discussing the topic during the work lunch hour. Thus, it is advantageous for employers to partner with in-house or community EAPs for dealing with workplace violence and intimate partner violence (Paludi and Paludi, 2000; Bryant, Eliach, & Green 1991; Rothman, Hathaway, Stidsen, & deVries, 2007). An EAP assists employees with dealing with non–work-related issues that interfere with their ability to perform their job (Smith & Mazin, 2004). EAPs provide short-term counseling on the telephone or in person as well as refer employees for help in the community. An EAP can be utilized to help women employees deal with the symptomatology of intimate partner violence reviewed above (Paludi & Paludi, 2000; Rothman, Hathaway, Stidsen, & deVries, 2007).

Recommendations for EAPs include helping women to develop a sense of trust and safety in the current work environment, understanding women's insecurity about their future, countering any sense of guilt about having caused the violence and/or not being able to prevent the violence, and increasing women's self-esteem (Paludi, Wilmot, & Speach, 2010). Information shared by EAPs also should include local shelters, impact of intimate partner violence on victims, impact of intimate partner violence on children, and cultural issues involved in reporting and not reporting the abuse (Bostock, Plupton, & Pratt, 2009).

CONCLUSION

The Partnership for Prevention (2002) reported that most employers do not have defined policies and procedures for dealing with intimate partner violence that spills over into the workplace. Smaller companies are less likely than larger companies to include a policy on intimate partner violence. Services that are most commonly offered by companies have included victim referral services, security precautions, and educational materials (e.g., posters, brochures). Roper's (2002) study of the Liz Claiborne survey of Fortune 1000 senior executives and managers indicated that victim resources were the only focus of these employers' attention to intimate partner violence, including emergency counseling services, employee benefits that covered the costs of medical assistance, and referrals to organizations that deal with intimate partner violence.

In order for these recommendations for prevention strategies to be successful, there must be support and initiative from the president of the organization. Without this commitment, the prevention strategies will not be effectively implemented, contributing to employees believing that the organization is not seriously committed to the issue of intimate partner violence and thus being silenced about their experiences with this abuse. Furthermore, as has been suggested in this chapter, dealing with intimate partner violence as a workplace issue must be based on a multidisciplinary team approach, including human resources, EAPs, security, managers, law enforcement, attorneys, and employees themselves (Lieber, 2011; Versola-Russo & Russo, 2009). Unions may also assist by supporting the company's intimate partner violence policy, facilitating training on intimate partner violence for new stewards/delegates, and ensuring that all employees have received the company's policy and have been trained on intimate partner violence (Paludi, Wilmot, & Speach, 2010).

Members of the Corporate Alliance to End Partner Violence have instituted various programs to bring awareness of intimate partner violence to employees. For example, Liz Claiborne features information about its commitment to the prevention of intimate partner violence on hand tags on garments that the company manufactures. Also included on the hand tags is the toll free number of the National Domestic Violence Hotline. In addition, Liz Claiborne instituted policies, procedures, and training programs on intimate partner violence. The company's EAP provides trained counselors on intimate partner violence 24 hours per day via an 800 number. Liz Claiborne also provides extended leave without pay and short-term paid leaves of absence for victims of intimate partner violence.

Allstate Insurance Company founded SAFE HANDS, a network for empowering women who are victims of intimate partner violence. This program offers direct services, including training programs and research on public awareness about intimate partner violence.

Kaiser Permanente has four components to its intimate violence program: screening and referral, a supportive work environment, on-site resources for employees, and community linkages. In addition, Kaiser Permanente developed its silentWitness project, which depicts stories from employees who are victims of intimate partner violence. The company has translated women's stories from English into Spanish and Cantonese. Kaiser Permanente's electronic medical record includes screening and assessment for intimate partner violence.

The Occupational Safety and Health Administration recommends that employers include preventative measures in their workplace violence management programs. Principles of effective prevention programs include the following:

a. Support by infrastructure and institutional commitment.
b. Proactive measures.
c. A workplace culture that does not foster a climate of violence.
d. Integrating legal, management, and psychological approaches.
e. Employees practicing the prevention plan.
f. Reevaluating the plan and revising it as necessary.
g. Strategic and targeted goals.

These organizations as well as others in the Corporate Alliance to End Partner Violence integrate the empirical research on intimate partner violence as a workplace issue in their prevention and reactive measures. They serve as models for other organizations that have the opportunity to use their power to create change in their companies as well as in society with respect to ending intimate partner violence. Intimate partner violence is not only a workplace issue but is also a human rights issue.

REFERENCES

American Bar Association Commission on Domestic Violence (1999). *A guide for employees: Domestic violence in the workplace.* Washington, DC: Author.

American Institute on Domestic Violence (2009). Domestic violence in the workplace statistics. Retrieved from http://www.cycsf.org/yawav/statistics.php.

Babcock, J., Miller, S. & Siard, C. (2003). Toward a typology of abusive women: Differences between partner-only and generally-violent women in the use of violence. *Psychology of Women Quarterly, 27,* 153–161,

Birns, B. (1999). Battered wives: Causes, effects and social change. In C. Forden, A. Hunter, & B. Birns (Eds.), *Readings in the psychology of women: Dimensions of the female experience* (pp. 328–339). Boston: Allyn & Bacon.

Black, D., & Newman, M. (2000). Children: Secondary victims of domestic violence. In A. Shalev et al. (Eds.), *International handbook of human responses to trauma* (pp. 129–138). New York: Plenum.

Bostock, J., Plumpton, M., & Pratt, R. (2009). Domestic violence against women: Understanding social processes and women's experiences. *Journal of Community and Applied Social Psychology, 19,* 95–110.

Bryant, V., Eliach, J. & Green, S. (1991). Adapting the traditional EAP model to effectively serve battered women in the workplace. *Employee Assistance Quarterly, 6,* 1–10.

Butts Stahly, G. (1999). Violence against women by male partners: Prevalence, outcomes and policy implications. *American Psychologist, 48,* 1077–1087.

Centers for Disease Control and Prevention (2008). Adverse health conditions and health risk behaviors associated with intimate partner violence. Retrieved on January 29, 2011, from http://www.cdc.gov/mmwr/preview/mmwrhtml/mm5705a1.htm.

Coleman, V. (1991). Violence in lesbian couples: A between groups comparison. Doctoral dissertation, California School of Professional Psychology, Los Angeles, 1990. *Dissertation Abstracts International 51,* 5634B.

Corporate Alliance to End Partner Violence (2005). CAEP news. Retrieved on January 30, 2011, from http://www.caepv.org/about/releasedetail.php?prID=89.

Corporate Alliance to End Partner Violence (2007). CEO and employee survey. Retrieved on January 30, 2011, from http://www.caepv.org/about/program_detail.php?refID=34.

Cunradi, C., Ames, G., & Moore, R. (2008). Prevalence and correlates of intimate partner violence among a sample of construction industry workers. *Journal of Family Violence, 23,* 101–112.

Feblinger, D. (2008). The impact of violence in the nursing workplace and women's lives. *Journal of Obstetric, Gynecologic, and Neonatal Nursing, 37,* 216–218.

Graham, D., & Rawlings, E. (1999). Observers' blaming of battered wives: Who, what, when, and why. In M. Paludi (Ed.), *The psychology of sexual victimization: A handbook* (pp. 55–94). Westport, CT: Greenwood.

Grothues, C., & Marmion, S. (2006). Dismantling the myths about intimate violence against women. In P. Lundberg-Love & S. Marmion (Eds.), *Intimate violence against women* (pp. 9–14). Westport, CT: Praeger.
Horne, S. (1999). Domestic violence in Russia. *American Psychologist, 54,* 55–61.
Kelloway, E., Barling, J., & Hurrell, J. (2006). *Handbook of workplace violence.* New York: Sage.
Knefel, A., & Bryant, C. (2004). Workplace as combat zone: Reconceptualizing occupational and organizational violence. *Deviant Behavior, 25,* 579–601.
Lemon, N. (2001). *Domestic violence law.* St. Paul, MN: West Group.
Lieber, L. (2011). HR's role in preventing workplace violence. *Employment Relations Today, 37,* 83–88.
Lloyd, S., & Taluc, N. (1999). The effects of male violence on female employment. *Violence Against Women, 5,* 370–392.
Lundberg-Love, P., & Marmion, S. (2006). *Intimate violence against women.* Westport, CT: Praeger.
Lundberg-Love, P., & Wilkerson, D. (2006). Battered women. In P. Lundberg-Love & S. Marmion (Eds.), *Intimate violence against women* (pp. 31–45). Westport, CT: Praeger.
Marmion, S., & Faulkner, D. (2006). Effects of class and culture on intimate partner violence. In P. Lundberg-Love & S. Marmion (Eds.), *Intimate violence against women* (pp. 131–143). Westport, CT: Praeger.
McHugh, M., & Frieze, I. (2006). Intimate partner violence. In F. Denmark, H. Krauss, E. Halpern, & J. Sechzer (Eds.), *Violence and exploitation against women and girls* (pp. 121–141). Boston: Blackwell.
McHugh, M., Livingston, N., & Frieze, I. (2008). Intimate partner violence: Perspectives on research and intervention. In F. Denmark & M. Paludi (Eds.), *Psychology of women: A handbook of issues and theories* (pp. 555–589). Westport, CT: Praeger.
Middelkoop, J, Gilhooley, J., Ruepp, N., Polikoski, R., & Paludi, M. (2008). Campus security recommendations for administrators to help prevent and deal with violence. In M. Paludi (Ed.), *Understanding and preventing campus violence* (pp. 234–235). Westport, CT: Praeger.
National Institute for Occupational Safety and Health (2010). *Occupational violence.* Retrieved on January 30, 2011, from www.niosh.gov.
Nydegger, R., Paludi, M., DeSouza, E., & Paludi, C. (2006). Incivility, sexual harassment and violence in the workplace. In M. Karsten (Ed.), *Gender, race and ethnicity in the workplace* (pp. 52–81). Westport, CT: Praeger.
Occupational Safety and Health Administration (2010). Workplace violence. Retrieved on January 30, 2011, from www.osha.org.
O'Leary, K., & Maiuro, R. (Eds.). (2001). *Psychological abuse in violent domestic relations.* New York: Springer.
Paludi, M. (2002). *The psychology of women* (2nd ed.). Upper Saddle River, NJ: Prentice Hall.
Paludi, M., & Barickman, R. (1998). *Sexual harassment, work, and education: A resource manual for prevention.* Albany: State University of New York Press.
Paludi, M., Nydegger, R., & Paludi, C. (2006). *Understanding workplace violence: A guide for managers and employees.* Westport, CT: Praeger.
Paludi, C., & Paludi, M. (2000, October). *Developing and enforcing an effective workplace policy statement, procedures, and training programs on domestic violence.* Paper presented at the Conference on Domestic Violence as a Workplace Concern: Legal, Psychological, Management, and Law Enforcement Perspectives, Nashua, NH.

Paludi, M., & Paludi, C. (2006). Integrating work/life: Resources for employees, employers, and human resource specialists. In M. Paludi & P. Neidermeyer (Eds.), *Work, life and family imbalance: How to level the playing field* (pp. 122–154). Westport, CT: Praeger.

Paludi, M., Paludi, C., & DeSouza, E. (Eds.). (2010). *Praeger handbook on understanding and preventing workplace discrimination.* Westport, CT: Praeger.

Paludi, M., Vaccariello, R., Graham, T., Smith, M., Allen-Dicker, K., Kasprzak, H., & White, C. (2006). Work/life integration: Impact on women's career, employment and family. In M. Paludi & P. Neidermeyer (Eds.), *Work, life and family imbalance: How to level the playing field* (pp. 21–36). Westport, CT: Praeger.

Paludi, M., Wilmot, J., & Speach, L. (2010). Intimate partner violence as a workplace concern: Impact on women's emotional and physical well-being and careers. In M. Paludi (Ed.), *Feminism and women's rights worldwide* (pp. 103–137). Westport, CT: Praeger.

Partnership for Prevention (2002). *Domestic violence and the workplace.* Washington, DC: Author.

Potoczniak, M., Murot, J., Crosbie-Burnett, M., & Potoczni, A. (2003). Legal and psychological perspectives on same-sex domestic violence. *Journal of Family Psychology, 17,* 252–259.

Probst, T., Estrada, A., & Brown, J. (2008). Harassment, violence and hate crimes in the workplace. In K. Thomas (Ed.), *Diversity resistance in organizations* (pp. 93–125). New York: Erlbaum.

Randel, J., & Wells, K. (2003). Corporate approaches to reducing intimate partner violence through workplace initiatives. *Clinical Occupation and Environmental Medicine, 3,* 821–841.

Rathus, J., & Feindler, E. (2004). *Assessment of partner violence: A handbook for researchers and practitioners.* Washington, DC: American Psychological Association.

Reeves, C., & O'Leary-Kelly, A. (2007). The effects and costs of intimate partner violence for work organizations. *Journal of Interpersonal Violence, 22,* 327–344.

Ridley, E. (2004). *Impact of Domestic Violence Offenders on Occupational Safety and Health: A Pilot Study.* Portland: Family Crisis Services, Maine Department of Labor.

Roper, A. (2002). *Corporate leaders on domestic violence awareness of the problem, how it's affecting their business, and what they're doing to address it.* New York: Liz Claiborne.

Rothman, E., Hathaway, J., Stidsen, A., & deVries, H. (2007). How employment helps female victims of intimate partner violence: A qualitative study. *Journal of Occupational Health Psychology, 12,* 136–143.

Sagrestano, L., Carroll, D., Rodriguez, A., & Nuwayhid, B. (2004). Demographic, psychological and relationship factors in domestic violence during pregnancy in a sample of low-income women of color. *Psychology of Women Quarterly, 28,* 309–322.

Schaffer, K., Casteel, C., & Kraus, J. (2002). A case-site/control-site study of workplace violent injury. *Journal of Occupational and Environmental Medicine, 44,* 1018–1026.

Smith, S., & Mazin, R. (2004). *The HR answer book.* New York: AMACOM.

Soroptimist International of the Americas (2007). *White paper: Domestic violence as a workplace concern.* Retrieved on June 22, 2009, from http://staging.soroptimist.org/whitepapers/wp_dv.html.

Stewart, M., & Kleiner, B. (1997). How to curb workplace violence. *Facilities, 15,* 5–11.

Straus, M., Gelles, R., & Steinmetz, S. (1980). *Behind closed doors: Violence in the American family.* Garden City, NY: Anchor Books.

Swanberg, J., & Logan, T. (2005). Domestic violence and employment: A qualitative study of the effects of domestic violence on women's employment. *Journal of Occupational and Health Psychology, 10,* 3–17.

Swanberg, J., & Logan, T. (2007). Intimate partner violence, employment and the workplaces: An interdisciplinary perspective. *Journal of Interpersonal Violence, 22,* 263–267.

Swanberg, J., Logan, T., & Macke, C. (2005). Intimate partner violence, employment and the workplace: Consequences and future directions. *Trauma, Violence, & Abuse, 6,* 286–312.

Swanberg, J., Macke, C., & Logan, T. (2006). Intimate partner violence, women, and work: Coping on the job. *Violence and Victims, 21,* 561–578.

Tjaden, P., & Thoennes, N. (2000). *Full report of the prevalence, incidence and consequences of violence against women: Findings from the National Violence Against Women Survey, NIJ/CDC.* U.S. Department of Justice. (NCJ 183781).

Tran, C., & DesJardins, K. (2000). Domestic violence in Vietnamese refugee and Korean immigrant communities. In J. Chin (Ed.), *Relationships among Asian American women* (pp. 261–285). Washington, DC: American Psychological Association.

Versola-Russo, J., & Russo, F. (2009). When domestic violence turns into workplace violence: Organizational impact and response. *Journal of Police Crisis Negotiations, 9,* 141–148.

Walker, L. (1999). Psychology and domestic violence around the world. *American Psychologist, 54,* 21–29.

Walker, L. (2006). Battered woman syndrome: Empirical findings. In F. Denmark, H. Krauss, E. Halpern, & J. Sechzer (Eds.), *Violence and exploitation against women and girls* (pp. 142–157). Boston: Blackwell.

Wetterstein, K., Rudolph, S., Paul, K., Gallagher, K., Trang, B., Adams, K., Graham, S., & Terrance, C. (2004). Freedom through self-sufficiency: A qualitative examination of the impact of violence on the working lives of women in shelters. *Journal of Counseling Psychology, 51,* 447–462.

Willman, S. (2007). *Too much, too long? Domestic violence in the workplace.* Testimony before the U.S. Senate Subcommittee on Employment and Workplace Safety, Washington, DC.

Worthington, K. (2000). Violence in the health care workplace. *American Journal of Nursing, 100,* 69–70.

Zorza, J. (2002). Battering. In J. Zorza (Ed.), *Violence against women.* Kingston, NJ: Civic Research Institute.

Chapter 6

The Effects of Sexism, Gender Microaggressions, and Other Forms of Discrimination on Women's Mental Health and Development

Kevin L. Nadal and Kristal Haynes

The United States is often characterized as being the land of opportunity and equality in which people of all races, ethnicities, genders, and religions as well as other groups would be treated equally and have the chance of achieving the American Dream. In many ways this depiction is true. People of color and women are now allowed to vote, own property, and attain an education. Women are entering the workforce at much higher numbers than before. People have the freedom to practice whichever religion they choose. People of all countries have become American citizens, and many have fulfilled aspirations that they may not have been able to accomplish in their homelands. Laws on federal and state levels prohibit people from being discriminated against because of their race, ethnicity, gender, or religion. Sexual harassment laws are now being enforced, and stricter punishments have been given to offenders who commit hate crimes that are committed because of a victim's religion, race, ethnicity, or sexual orientation. And as a final point, all children of any social class or background have access to education.

Despite these truths, there is also a contrasting argument that the United States does not provide equal opportunities to all groups. Depending on social class, race, ethnicity, gender, sexual orientation, or ability, people may not have the same privileges, access to resources, or opportunities as others, which then may affect their ability to thrive. A brief look at some of the economic, employment, and educational disparities that affect people of color and women may support this statement. According to the U.S. Equal Employment Opportunity Commission (2003), 85% of the Fortune 500 CEOs are men, and 97% of them are White. Moreover, the U.S. Census Bureau (2007) reports that people of color and White women do not make as much money as White men. There has only been one U.S. president of color, and there has yet to be a female president. People of color generally tend to enter and graduate from college at smaller rates than Whites, and women are underrepresented in a number of fields, including business, science, academia, and politics. If women account for approximately half the population of the United States and people of color are projected to become one-third of the total American population, why do these disparities in income, employment, and education exist? Perhaps people of color do not have the same opportunities as Whites, and women do not have the same opportunities as men. Moreover, perhaps these groups experience discrimination and other obstacles that may prevent them from reaching their optimal success.

In spite of some of these institutional disparities, perhaps the decrease in interpersonal discrimination over the years is what has painted the picture that the United States offers equality for all. Over the past two decades or so, it has become socially unacceptable for people to express prejudice in public and in social circles. In present times, most Americans would view blatantly racist acts and racial or ethnic hate crimes as unacceptable and appalling (Nadal, 2008). In fact, many individuals have adopted a culture of political correctness (in which individuals are careful to use nonoffensive language in order to be sensitive to diversity). People, especially White Americans, may genuinely believe that they are good people and that they treat others of different racial groups the same. Thus, individuals may not engage in overtly racist acts themselves and therefore may believe that discrimination no longer exists.

However, while overtly prejudiced acts may be less acceptable in the United States, some have argued that racism and other forms of discrimination still occur in everyday life but take on more subtle forms (Sue, 2010). For example, although sexual harassment is outlawed, it is common for women to face institutional and subtle sexism in the workplace. As aforementioned, women do not get paid as much as men and are also not promoted as often as men, and gender still affects how women are treated in the workplace. Two examples that may demonstrate this concept include a female employee who is not invited to a social outing (e.g., a baseball game or drinks with male coworkers) or a female top executive who is asked to engage in traditional gender roles (e.g., coordinating the office party when this is clearly not part of her high-ranking job). In both situations, these women may not be experiencing explicit sexism, but perhaps they are being treated differently because of their gender. Furthermore, women may encounter more covert sexism that may not meet the requirements of sexual harassment; thus, they may not report such behaviors when they occur. For example, if a female employee overhears a male coworker making jokes that are subtly sexist, she may experience distress and be offended, but she may not know how to address the situation. She does not think that her coworker was intentionally trying to be sexist, and she does not think that it is significant enough to report the incident to human resources. Plus, she knows that she runs the risk of being dismissed as being paranoid or overly sensitive.

These types of subtle slights and uncomfortable situations have been labeled as microaggressions. Microaggressions are brief and commonplace daily verbal, behavioral, and environmental indignities (often unconscious and unintentional) that communicate hostile, derogatory, or invalidating messages toward people of marginalized groups (Nadal, 2008; Sue, Bucceri, et al., 2007; Sue, 2010). There has been an increase in academic literature that has described the types of microaggressions that individuals experience and the impacts that such incidents have on individuals' mental health. Microaggression literature has focused on experiences of various groups, including people of color (e.g., Rivera, Forquer, & Rangel, 2010; Sue, Bucceri, et al., 2007; Sue, Nadal, et al., 2008; Watkins, LaBarrie, & Appio, 2010); lesbian, gay, bisexual, and transgender populations (e.g., Nadal, Rivera, & Corpus, 2010); and women (e.g., Capodilupo et al., 2010; Nadal, 2010; Nadal, Hamit, Lyons, Weinberg, & Corman, in press). The empirical literature suggests that microaggressions often lead to an array of emotions for these individuals, including anger, sadness, belittlement, frustration, and alienation, and that the cumulative nature of these microaggressions therefore may potentially lead to mental health problems, including depression, anxiety, and trauma (for a review, see Sue, 2010).

Previous research on microaggressions has indicated that victims of such incidents react in a number of ways (Nadal, Hamit, et al., in press; Nadal, Wong, et al., in press; Sue, Capodilupo, & Holder, 2008). Emotionally they may respond with anger, sadness, guilt, or frustration. Behaviorally they react by confronting the individual, passively walking away, or avoiding certain people or environments. Cognitively, some individuals describe how microaggressions have led them to become resilient, while others report learning to accept microaggressions as part of their everyday lives. Many authors (e.g., Nadal, 2008, 2010; Sue, 2010; Sue & Sue, 2008) have argued that microaggressions may cause more harm toward individuals than overt forms of racism. Because microaggressions are often dismissed, ignored, invalidated, or viewed as innocuous, the victim of such an incident may feel paranoid, hypersensitive, or isolated. On the other hand, an individual who experiences an overt form of discrimination may feel more able to turn to others for support, may be able to label the act as discriminatory, and may have the opportunity to externalize any negative feelings about the incident and the perpetrator.

The current chapter will focus specifically on women's experiences of microaggressions and the impact of such experiences on their mental health. First, a review of the literature will examine the various types of microaggressions that women experience as well as the other types of sexism that they may encounter in their everyday lives. Next, we will discuss how gender microaggressions and sexism may negatively impact women's mental health, self-esteem, and identity development. Finally, we will examine how other microaggressions impact women with intersectional identities (particularly women of color and lesbian and bisexual women).

GENDER MICROAGGRESSIONS AND OTHER FORMS OF SEXISM

Nadal (2010, p. 156) defines gender microaggressions as "brief and commonplace daily verbal, behavioral, and environmental indignities that communicate hostile, derogatory, or negative sexist slights and insults toward women." In a qualitative study by Capodilupo et al. (2010), female participants described the various types of microaggressions that they experience in their everyday lives, naming incidents that could be classified into several categories: sexual objectification, assumptions of traditional gender roles, second-class citizenship, assumptions of inferiority, sexist language, denial of reality of sexism, denial of individual sexism, and environmental microaggressions. Sexual objectification refers to instances in which women are sexualized or denigrated for men's pleasure; for example, a woman is catcalled as she walks down the street, or a man subtly glares at a woman's breast. Assumptions of traditional gender roles signifies incidents in which women are expected to adhere to traditional roles. This can be demonstrated by a woman being questioned if she does not have any children or by a female employee who is assumed to take care of household chores at her workplace. Second-class citizenship refers to instances in which men receive preferential treatment; for instance, one participant described how male sports teams at her school received better equipment than female sports teams. Assumptions of inferiority is a category that describes experiences in which women are believed to be less intellectual or less physically capable of doing certain things (e.g., a woman who is assumed to not be a good leader or a man who assumes that a woman could not carry a box on her own). Sexist language refers to encounters in which women are belittled through jokes, statements, and other invalidating forms of verbal communication (e.g., being called a bitch). Denial of reality of sexism refers to experiences in which women are invalidated and dismissed when they identify the sexism that they still experience in their lives. Denial of individual sexism occurs when a man who is confronted on his sexist behavior dismisses his biases. Finally, environmental microaggressions are subtle forms of discrimination that are experienced through various systems and environments. Examples include when women notice that there are no female leaders in their companies and when women are sexualized or denigrated through the media.

These categories of gender microaggressions align closely with much of the previous literature that focuses on sexism. Traditionally when laypeople describe the term "sexism," they are referring to explicit, chauvinistic, and misogynistic behaviors that were very commonplace 20 years ago. While such sexism still exists, there are additional forms of sexism that may or may not fit the stereotypical definition. These include overt sexism (Swim & Cohen, 1997), covert sexism (Swim & Cohen, 1997), subtle sexism (Swim, Mallett, and Stagnor, 2004); benevolent sexism (Glicke & Fiske, 2001), and hostile sexism (Glicke & Fiske, 2001).

Swim and Cohen (1997) have labeled three types of sexism: overt sexism, covert sexism, and subtle sexism. Overt sexism refers to the old-fashioned sexism that women encounter and that is often easier to identify. For example, sexual harassment could be defined as overt sexism because these behaviors that occur in the workplace fit criteria that are identifiably sexist and are usually conscious and intentional by the perpetrator. Covert sexism occurs when unequal and harmful actions are committed in unconscious, unintentional, or hidden ways. In these types of cases, men may not intentionally or consciously hope to offend the women through their behavior; however, their behavior may communicate a hurtful message. Swim et al. (2004) describe subtle sexism as verbal or physical behaviors that may go unnoticed because they are often viewed as normal and behaviors that are not out of the ordinary. This can be demonstrated by an instance in which a female physician who is working at a hospital is assumed to be a nurse or when a high-ranking female executive is presumed to be a secretary. Another form of subtle sexism may include written documents when the word "he" is assumed to apply to both men and women.

Glick and Fiske (2001) describe two other forms of sexism that exist: benevolent sexism and hostile sexism. Benevolent sexism is defined as "a favorable, chivalrous ideology that offers protection and affection to women who embrace conventional roles," while hostile sexism is defined as animosity toward women who are seen to minimize men's power (p. 109). With benevolent sexism, men are usually well intended and believe that they are being chivalrous and polite; however, their verbal or physical behaviors may communicate messages that women should maintain traditional general roles. For instance, when a man helps a woman carrying a box when she did not show any distress or ask for help, he may unintentionally communicate his subconscious or unconscious bias that women are physically weak or incapable. With hostile sexism, men may be conscious and intentional in their biases toward women. An example may include a situation in which a male employee is threatened by a female supervisor's power and therefore belittles her capabilities to her or in front of others.

There are many ways that these five types of sexism are related to gender microaggressions, with the driving similarity involving the intention and consciousness of the behavior. Both covert sexism and subtle sexism fit well with several of the aforementioned examples of microaggressions, particularly with the assumptions of traditional gender roles (e.g., expecting a woman to complete household chores) or the assumptions of inferiority (e.g., presuming a woman to be physically weak). These types of experiences, while unintentional and unconscious, send harmful messages that women are supposed to maintain traditional gender roles or are physically or intellectually inferior. Examples of benevolent sexism may actually be forms of microaggressions because such behavior is well intentioned and conscious, without the enactor recognizing that what he perceives as chivalrous may actually be offensive to women. Finally, some forms of overt sexism or hostile sexism may be defined as gender microaggressions. For example, when a man objectifies a woman through sexist language or catcalling or when he belittles his female supervisor's qualifications or skills, he may be conscious and deliberate of his behavior, yet he may not be malicious in his intentions.

INFLUENCES OF SEXISM ON MENTAL HEALTH AND DEVELOPMENT

Regardless of how such sexism is labeled, it is important to recognize that such discrimination may have deleterious impacts on women's mental health and development. Previous literature has reported that women are susceptible to an array of mental health risks that their male counterparts may not experience. When women are objectified and experience sexism, they may become depressed, develop low self-esteem, or experience sexual dysfunction (Fredrickson & Roberts, 1997; Hill & Fischer, 2008; Kozee, Tylka, Augustus-Horvath, and Denchik, 2007). When women are expected to adhere to traditional gender roles, they may develop faulty cognitions, which may lead to depression, self-doubt, helplessness, passivity, and lower self-esteem (Sands, 1998). Furthermore, because women are objectified in society, many may develop eating disorders and body image issues (Kozee et al., 2007). Perhaps the unrealistic expectations of women's bodies in the media may lead to the increase of these eating disorders and may explain why eating disorders are continually on the rise for young girls (Sinclair, 2006; Stice & Bearman, 2001). One meta-analysis found that 40% of newly identified cases of anorexia are in young women 15–19 years old (Hoek & van Hoeken, 2003), while a well-known study discovered that 42% of 1st- through 3rd-grade girls in their sample want to be thinner (Collins, 1991). Thus, it is important to address sexism in the environment (e.g., the media), as well as sexism that is perpetuated interpersonally, as these types of sexism may lead to various mental health (and even physical health) problems (Sinclair, 2006; Stice & Bearman, 2001).

Sexism may also have an influence on women's gender role formation, which may also affect their mental health and development. Research has demonstrated that infants as young as 10 months old can begin to associate certain objects with different genders (i.e., they can identify trucks as being related to boys and dolls as being connected to girls). Furthermore, toddlers (around 18–24 months of age) can use and understand gendered words in their vocabulary (Martin & Ruble, 2010; Miller, Lurye, Zosuls, & Ruble, 2009). While these researchers argue that children exhibit gendered behavior prior to age 2, socialization theorists attribute gendered behavior to children actively seeking knowledge about their roles in society. The more information children receive about their respective gender category (which is usually in plentitude), the more they try to behave in accordance with their prescribed gender identity (Martin & Ruble, 2010).

When children develop certain cognitive abilities, they are also able to perceive differences between the sexes (and subsequent judgments about those differences). Brown and Bigler (2005) offer a developmental model of children's ability to perceive discrimination, stating that many children are familiar with the meaning of discrimination by age 10. Furthermore, these authors maintain that children recognize how gender discrimination is marked by differences in social status and salient aspects of one's identity. On the whole, children perceive discrimination to occur rather frequently, and as age increases children seem to better understand that the endorsement of stereotypes is linked to discrimination (Brown & Bigler, 2005; McKown & Weinstein, 2003).

Brown and Bigler's (2005) model set out to outline both the cognitive and situational factors that influence children's perceptions of discrimination. It was concluded that children must have a good grasp of cultural cognition or be culturally aware of the social meaning of gender. Additionally, children must have developed social perspective taking, which implies that they can grasp and recognize the thinking of others around them (Brown and Bigler, 2005; Quintana, 2008). Certain situational factors must be salient in order for children to recognize that the discrimination they are experiencing is based on their gender category. For instance, a young girl experiencing what can be categorized as a sexist event must be aware that she is the target of discrimination, must understand the motivation or intention of the actor(s) committing the derogatory act, must be able to compare this type of discrimination to other possible forms of discrimination, and must understand the relevance of stereotypical information to this interaction (Brown & Bigler). If children are able to recognize discrimination at a young age, such experiences have the ability to shape their developmental trajectory from that point onward. For example, through understanding racism and discrimination, young children of color may learn negative messages about their racial or ethnic groups, which may then influence their self-concept and social development. Similarly, sexism may influence little girls' impressions of themselves as well as their perceptions of their capabilities, which may then impact their self-esteem and their ability to succeed.

Martin and Ruble (2010) argue that from a very early age, children can also decipher differences in societally recognized power between men and women, understanding that society organizes its practices around gender. Furthermore, Miller et al. (2009) argue that children tend to hold very strict stereotypes about male and female behavior, leaving little room for individual variability. One study found that children tend to "punish" other children who deviate from sex role norms, children are able to recognize individuals who enforce these gender role rules more harshly than others, and children who dislike the harsh enforcers are more likely to stick closely to same-sex playmates (Martin and Ruble). It is unclear if this behavior stems from in-group admiration or the need to degrade the out-group, which would be an explanation according to intergroup relations literature. Nonetheless, it is possible that little girls during this age may attribute males as being more superior to females, which may then influence their views about women and power.

Furthermore, gender-based expectations are cited as deterring women from their optimal social, personal, and vocational development. Both girls and boys are embedded in a culture with high gender role expectations that are taught (explicitly and implicitly) by many sources and internalized through time. These gender role expectations then influence their identity development as well as many other aspects of their lives. Some examples of the ways that gender roles impact an individual's everyday experiences include one's abilities and perceptions in regard to household chores (e.g., girls are taught to cook and clean, while boys are taught to rake leaves or take out the garbage), their choice of clothing (e.g., girls are taught to wear dresses and like the color pink, while men are taught to wear pants and like the color blue), and even their everyday behaviors (e.g., girls are taught that it is acceptable to cry or show emotion, while boys are taught otherwise).

Several authors have also found that strict gender-based expectations impact self-concept and career options for girls through adolescence and beyond (Steffens, Jelenec, & Noack, 2010; Leaper & Brown, 2008). The frequency and pervasiveness of negative societal stereotypes about women (particularly regarding math and science) may cause girls to develop a negative academic self-concept regarding their math abilities. Such negative messages (which are communicated by parents, teachers, classmates, and the media) may also subconsciously influence a young girl's lack of desire to pursue a career in mathematics or the natural sciences (Steffens et al., 2010). This argument supports the introductory hypothesis that sexism and other forms of discrimination are in fact directly related to educational, economic, and vocational disparities.

One demonstration of how gender role expectations may influence career choice involves a speech by former Harvard University president Lawrence Summer in 2005. When discussing the lack of representation of women in the fields of math and science, he suggested that the disparity is due to the notion that females are not inclined in naturally logical-mathematical thinking as compared to the male population (Summers, 2005). His comments drew a firestorm from those who had taken offense with the sexist nature of his speech, arguing that women who expressed any interest in math and science would not receive the support or resources they needed in an institution that endorsed sexist rhetoric. While Summers's intentions may not have been to be insulting or hurtful, his words represented how unconscious biases may indeed lead to microaggressive invalidations and emotionally distressing outcomes for people of marginalized groups.

The identity development of girls is also highly affected by their experiences throughout adolescence. From the onset of puberty and the flourishing desire for romantic partners, sexual objectification becomes a growing concern for girls at this age. Objectification theory suggests that society tends to regard women's bodies as objects much more so than men's bodies, as evidenced by gazing patterns and sexually evaluative remarks being targeted toward women on a much more frequent basis (Frederickson & Roberts, 1997). Objectification is a symptom of a society that continues to build a power gap between males and females and seeks to justify such a system (Jost, Banaji, & Nosek, 2004). Female bodies are thought of as boosts to product sales, commodities to be traded, edited, and fantasized about.

According to objectification theory, women experience moments of disembodiment every day as they constantly think about how they feel in their skin and how the outside world will evaluate their physical appearance as well. They begin to internalize a desire to fit societal ideals regarding female body image and monitor their looks to a great degree (Lindberg, Grabe, & Hyde, 2007). Pubertal development for a girl may bring episodes of unwanted sexual attention in addition to this heightened sense of needing to conform to cultural body standards. In a number of studies internalized belief in objectification during adolescence and in adulthood has been linked to depression, anxiety, and disordered eating (Tolman, Impett, Tracy, & Michael, 2006; Lindberg et al., 2007; Hurt et al., 2007).

Conversely, not caring about strict gender roles and not being exposed to critical thinking (i.e., exposure to feminism) may moderate or mediate the ability to perceive sexism and its psychological impact (Leaper & Brown, 2008). Leaper & Brown (2008) hypothesized that girls who were unhappy with gender roles and girls who were exposed to feminism would be more likely to report sexual harassment. Using hierarchical regression, the authors looked at sexual harassment, academic sexism, and athletic sexism, controlling for race and socioeconomic status. The model was significant, and girls who were exposed to feminism in the media and who already held more egalitarian views about gender roles reported more harassment. Similarly, girls who were discontent with gender roles and who did not feel that they fit a typical female role also reported more harassment. Thus, exposure to feminism and education about gender roles may lead to women voicing their discontent with sexism and harassment instead of internalizing messages of inferiority or objectification.

Experiences with sexism may also influence a woman's identity development as a feminist or her ability to internalize sexist messages. Downing and Roush (1985) proposed a model of feminist identity development to demonstrate how women learn to achieve a positive feminist identity by accepting, grappling with, and processing their feelings about sexism and gender discrimination. Similar to other models exploring racial and sexual identity, Downing and Roush's model is a five-stage identity development model that highlights nonlinear and nonsequential stages and individual progression:

Stage 1. Passive acceptance occurs when a woman is oblivious to sexism and/or denies that individual or institutional sexism exists. This may be exemplified by a woman who allows men to treat her in mysogynistic ways, who denies that sexism impacts her everyday life, or who believes that men are superior intellectually or physically.

Stage 2. Revelation is when a woman becomes aware of sexism (e.g., through experiencing sexual harassment or studying sexism in a women's studies course). This stage usually leads to conflicting feelings of anger and guilt in which the woman wonders how she was ever blind to sexism.

Stage 3. Embeddedness-emanation occurs when women develop close emotional connections with other women and form a sisterhood or support system. Women may turn to each other so that they can feel affirmed in their new identities and feel validated with others who recognize sexism in the same ways that they do.

Stage 4. Synthesis occurs when an individual learns to value being a woman through transcending traditional sex roles and valuing men individually instead of stereotypically.

Stage 5. Active commitment involves the translation of an integrated identity into an identity whereby the woman is moved to meaningful and effective action.

A woman's feminist identity status may greatly influence her mental health and identity development. One study found that when women have a less-developed feminist identity, they may be less likely to recognize microaggressions in their everyday lives (Capodilupo et al., 2010). Thus, if a woman maintains an identity that is similar to Stage 1 (passive acceptance), it is likely that she may ignore gender microaggressions or even view such experiences as complimentary or positive. However, in upholding this worldview, she may internalize sexist messages and gender role expectations, which may cause her to become depressed, develop low self-esteem, or develop body image issues. On the contrary, if a woman holds a worldview that is similar to Stages 4 or 5, she may learn to feel empowered as a woman, which may then increase her self-esteem and other protective factors against mental health problems.

INFLUENCES OF INTERSECTIONAL IDENTITIES

Many women may experience additional stressors and experience different types of microaggressions due to their other marginalized identities. Women of color may experience microaggressions that are based on their gender, their race, or some combination of both, while lesbian and bisexual women may have similar encounters based on the intersections of their gender and sexual orientation. Both racial microaggressions and sexual orientation/transgender microaggressions have been found to have negative mental health impacts on people of color and lesbian, gay, bisexual, and transgendered (LGBT) individuals (for a review, see Sue, 2010). However, when an individual belongs to two (or more) marginalized groups, she or he may experience even more difficulties with microaggressions. Not only might the individual have difficulty in identifying a microaggression, but she or he may have the stressor of identifying whether the microaggression is based on one of her or his identities or both. Furthermore, because of their multiple identities, it then becomes possible that there will be the potential for an increased amount of experiences with microaggressions.

As with gender microaggressions, there are several types of racial microaggressions that exist (see Sue, Capodilupo, et al., 2007; Sue, 2010). Some of these include the categories of "alien in one's own land" and "assumption of criminality." The alien in one's own land category refers to instances where people of color are presumed to be foreigners or immigrants regardless of their actual history or immigration status. For example, many Asian Americans and Latinos are often asked where they are from. When one of these individuals responds with "California" or "New York," the enactor of the microaggression may ask again where the individual is from because the enactor does not believe that the individual would be American. Another example of a racial microaggression includes the category of assumption of criminality. These incidents occur when someone assumes that a person of color would be a criminal when she or he did not give any real reason for another to believe that. For example, when an African American enters an elevator and a White individual already on the elevator moves away (or clutches one's purse or wallet), she or he is communicating a bias that African Americans are dangerous or would steal.

Women of color may experience an array of microaggressions based on their respective racial or ethnic identities. For example, in a study of Asian Americans, women reported feeling exoticized by men, particularly expressing how they often felt that men viewed them as trophy wives or girlfriends (Sue, Bucceri, et al., 2008). Rivera, Forquer, and Rangel (2010) found that Latina women experienced microaggressions in which people, particularly men, assumed them to be spicy and sassy. Finally, studies with African Americans reported that Black women encountered different types of microaggressions involving their hair (e.g., someone commenting on their hair as being either different or unprofessional) or assumptions of stereotypes (e.g., that they would be the angry Black woman).

Similarly, LGBT people may experience microaggressions based on their sexual orientation or transgender identity (see Nadal et al., 2010). Two examples of these categories of microaggressions include discomfort/disapproval of LGBT experience and the assumption of sexual pathology or abnormality. The former category refers to experiences in which individuals consciously or unconsciously express their disapproval of LGBT people; examples may include subtle or glaring stares when same-sex couples show public displays of affection or a parent who tries to convince her or his child to be heterosexual. Both send denigrating messages that there is something deviant or wrong about being an LGBT individual. The latter category refers to incidents in which LGBT people are presumed to be sexually deviant or malicious. For example, when people express verbally and behaviorally that they assume that a gay man has HIV/AIDS or is a child molester or that bisexual people are promiscuous, they communicate hurtful messages to the LGBT people who experience them.

Because of their dual identities, it may be common for lesbian and bisexual women to undergo microaggressions that may be based on their gender, their sexual orientation, or both. For example, when a man asks a lesbian or bisexual woman to engage in group sex, he may be exoticizing her based on her gender, her sexuality, or some combination of both. Similarly, if a lesbian or gay woman is refused service or is treated as a second-class citizen, it is unclear whether she is being discriminated against because she is a woman or because of her sexual orientation. Thus, an increase in microaggressions based on multiple identities may cause stressors that individuals with singular identities may not encounter.

Additionally, people with multiple identities may encounter unique psychological stressors that their counterparts may not face. First, when people belong to more than one group, they may often feel compelled to choose one identity over the other. For example, in a classroom discussion involving diversity, a woman of color may often feel compelled to represent her racial group or her gender but not both. Second, sometimes people may not feel fully comfortable in both of their communities at any given time. Because of the many dynamics that can occur between groups (e.g., communities of color that are overtly or covertly homophobic or heterosexist, LGBT communities that are overtly or covertly racist, women's social circles that ignore racial or LGBT issues), individuals may not feel that they fully belong in any of their respective groups. For example, a Latina lesbian might feel both connected and disconnected in her Latino community (where perhaps she is one of a few LGBT people) as well as feel both connected and disconnected in her LGBT community (where perhaps she is one of a few women of color). The experience of having multiple identities may result in potential mental health outcomes, including identity confusion, self-esteem issues, or emotional trauma.

CONCLUSION

This chapter examined the myriad ways that a woman's experiences with sexism, gender microaggressions, and other forms of discrimination may have an impact on her mental health or development. It is important to recognize that sexism (and other forms of discrimination) are still present in contemporary society so that measures can be taken to minimize and eliminate such discrimination altogether. As discussed in the chapter, discrimination can lead to an array of mental health outcomes, particularly for women. Some of these problems include depression, eating disorders, and body image issues, which all may also affect physical health problems. Experiences with sexism and gender microaggressions may also negatively impact an individual's social and personal development. Women may learn to internalize sexism and gender role expectations throughout their lives, which may then lead to low self-esteem, self-hatred, and difficulties in developing a healthy identity. Thus, it is crucial for educators, helping professionals, and people in general to address sexism on individual, group, and institutional levels in order to promote the most favorable mental health experiences for women.

REFERENCES

Brown, C., & Bigler, R. (2005). Children's perceptions of discrimination: A developmental model. *Child Development, 76,* 533–553.

Capodilupo, C. M., Nadal, K. L., Corman, L., Hamit, S., Lyons, O., & Weinberg, A. (2010). The manifestation of gender microaggressions. In D. W. Sue (Ed.), *Microaggressions and marginality: Manifestation, dynamics, and impact* (pp. 193–216). New York: Wiley.

Collins, M. E. (1991). Body figure perceptions and preferences among pre-adolescent children. *International Journal of Eating Disorders, 10,* 199–208.

Downing, N. E., & Roush, K. L. (1985). From passive acceptance to active commitment: A model of feminist identity development for women. *Counseling Psychologist, 13,* 695–709.

Fredrickson, B. L., & Roberts, T. (1997). Objectification theory: Toward understanding women's lived experiences and mental health risks. *Psychology of Women Quarterly, 21,* 173–206.

Glick, P., & Fiske, S. T. (2001) An ambivalent alliance: Hostile and benevolent sexism as complementary justifications for gender inequality. *American Psychologist, 56,* 109–118.

Hill, M. S., & Fischer, A. R. (2008). Examining objectification theory: Lesbian and heterosexual women's experiences with sexual- and self-objectification. *Counseling Psychologist, 36,* 745–776.

Hoek, H. W., & van Hoeken, D. (2003). Review of the prevalence and incidence of eating disorders. *International Journal of Eating Disorders, 34,* 383–396.

Hurt, M. M., Nelson, J. A., Turner, D. L., Haines, M. E., Ramsey, L. R., Erchull, M. J., & Liss, M. (2007). Feminism: What is it good for? Feminine norms and objectification as the link between feminist identity and clinically relevant outcomes. *Sex Roles, 57,* 355–363.

Jost, J. T., Banaji, M. R., & Nosek, B. A. (2004). A decade of system justification theory: Accumulated evidence of conscious and unconscious bolstering of the status quo. *Political Psychology, 25,* 881–919.

Kozee, H. B., Tylka, T. L., Augustus-Horvath, C. L., and Denchik, A. (2007) Development of psychometric evaluation of the Interpersonal Sexual Objectification Scale. *Psychology of Women Quarterly, 31,* 176–189.

Leaper, C., & Brown, C. (2008). Perceived experiences with sexism among adolescent girls. *Child Development, 79,* 685–704.

Lindberg, S. M., Grabe, S., & Hyde, J. (2007). Gender, pubertal development, and peer sexual harassment predict objectified body consciousness in early adolescence. *Journal of Research on Adolescence, 17,* 723–742.

Martin, C., & Ruble, D. N. (2010). Patterns of gender development. *Annual Review of Psychology, 61,* 353–381.

McKown, C., & Weinstein, R. (2003). The development and consequences of stereotype consciousness in middle childhood. *Child Development, 74,* 498–515.

Miller, C., Lurye, L. E., Zosuls, K. M., & Ruble, D. N. (2009). Accessibility of gender stereotype domains: Developmental and gender differences in children. *Sex Roles, 60,* 870–881.

Nadal, K. L. (2008). Preventing racial, ethnic, gender, sexual minority, disability, and religious microaggressions: Recommendations for promoting positive mental health. *Prevention in Counseling Psychology: Theory, Research, Practice and Training, 2,* 22–27.

Nadal, K. L. (2010). Gender microaggressions and women: Implications for mental health. In M. A. Paludi (Ed.), *Feminism and women's rights worldwide: Vol. 2. Mental and physical health* (pp. 155–175). Santa Barbara, CA: Praeger.

Nadal, K. L., Hamit, S., Lyons, O., Weinberg, A., & Corman, L., (in press). Gender microaggressions: Perceptions, processes, and coping mechanisms of women. In M. A. Paludi (Ed). *Managing diversity in today's workplace.* Santa Barbara, CA: Praeger.

Nadal, K. L., Rivera, D. P., & Corpus, M. J. H. (2010) Sexual orientation and transgender microaggressions in everyday life: Experiences of lesbians, gays, bisexuals, and transgender individuals. In D. W. Sue (Ed.), *Microaggressions and marginality: Manifestation, dynamics, and impact* (pp. 217–240). New York: Wiley.

Nadal, K. L., Wong, Y., Issa, M., Meterko, V., Leon, J., & Wideman, M. (in press). Sexual orientation microaggressions: Processes and coping mechanisms for lesbian, gay, and bisexual individuals. *Journal of LGBT Issues in Counseling.*

Quintana, S. M. (2008). Racial perspective taking ability: Developmental, theoretical, and empirical trends. In S. M. Quintana, C. McKown, S. M. Quintana, & C. McKown (Eds.), *Handbook of race, racism, and the developing child* (pp. 16–36). Hoboken, NJ: Wiley.

Rivera, D. P., Forquer, E. E., & Rangel, R. (2010). Microaggressions and the life experience of Latina/o Americans. In D. W. Sue (Ed.), *Microaggressions and marginality: Manifestation, dynamics, and impact* (pp. 59–83). New York: Wiley.

Sands, T. (1998). Feminist counseling and female adolescents: Treatment strategies for depression. *Journal of Mental Health Counseling, 20,* 42–54.

Sinclair, S. L. (2006). Object lessons: A theoretical and empirical study of objectified body consciousness in women. *Journal of Mental Health Counseling, 28,* 48–68.

Steffens, M. C., Jelenec, P., & Noack, P. (2010). On the leaky math pipeline: Comparing implicit math-gender stereotypes and math withdrawal in female and male children and adolescents. *Journal of Educational Psychology, 102,* 947–963.

Stice, E., & Bearman, S. K. (2001). Body-image and eating disturbances prospectively predict increases in depressive symptoms in adolescent girls: A growth curve analysis. *Developmental Psychology, 37,* 597–607.

Sue, D. W. (2010). *Microaggressions in everyday life: Race, gender, and sexual orientation* New York: Wiley.

Sue, D. W., Bucceri, J. M., Lin, A. I., Nadal, K. L., & Torino, G. C. (2007). Racial microaggressions and the Asian American experience. *Cultural Diversity and Ethnic Minority Psychology, 13,* 72–81.

Sue, D. W., Capodilupo, C. M., & Holder, A. M. B. (2008). Racial microaggressions in the life experience of Black Americans. *Professional Psychology: Research and Practice, 39,* 329–336.

Sue, D. W., Capodilupo, C. M., Torino, G. C., Bucceri, J. M., Holder, A. M., Nadal, K. L., & Esquilin, M. E. (2007). Racial microaggressions in everyday life: Implications for counseling. *American Psychologist, 62,* 271–286.

Sue, D. W., Nadal, K. L., Capodilupo, C. M., Lin, A. I., Rivera, D. P., & Torino, G. C. (2008). Racial microaggressions against Black Americans: Implications for counseling. *Journal of Counseling and Development, 8,* 330–338.

Sue, D. W., & Sue, D. (2008). *Counseling the culturally diverse: Theory and practice* (5th ed.). New York: Wiley.

Summers, L. (2005). Remarks at NBER Conference on diversifying the science & engineering workforce. Harvard University website, Office of the President, January 14. http://www.nber.org/~sewp/events/2005.01.14/Agenda-1-14-05-WEB.htm.

Swim, J. K., & Cohen, L. L. (1997). Overt, covert, and subtle sexism: A comparison between the attitudes toward women and modern sexism scales. *Psychology of Women Quarterly, 21,* 103–118.

Swim, J. K., Mallett, R., & Stagnor, C. (2004) Understanding subtle sexism: Detection and use of sexist language. *Sex Roles, 51,* 117–128.

Tolman, D. L., Impett, E. A., Tracy, A. J., & Michael, A. (2006). Looking good, sounding good: Femininity ideology and adolescent girls' mental health. *Psychology of Women Quarterly, 30,* 85–95.

U.S. Census Bureau (2007). Current population survey, table PINC-01: Selected characteristics of people, by total money income in 2006, work experience in 2006, race, Hispanic origin, and sex. Retrieved on September 25, 2010, from http://pubdb3.census.gov/macro/032007/perinc/new01_001.htm.

U.S. Equal Employment Opportunity Commission (2003). Women of color: Their employment in the private sector. Retrieved on May 24, 2010, from http://archive.eeoc.gov/stats/reports/womenofcolor/womenofcolor.pdf.

Watkins, N. L., LaBarrie, T. L., & Appio, L. M. (2010). Black undergraduates' experience with perceived racial microaggressions in predominantly White colleges and universities. In D. W. Sue (Ed.), *Microaggressions and marginality: Manifestation, dynamics, and impact* (pp. 25–58). New York: Wiley.

Chapter 7

Sexual Orientation Hate Crimes and the Experiences of LGBT Women

Katie E. Griffin and David A. Schuberth

Humbolt, Nebraska, December 24, 1993: A 21-year-old transsexual man is sexually assaulted and murdered after reporting the attack.

Jasper, Texas, June 7, 1998: A 49-year-old African American man is chained by his ankles to a pickup truck and dragged for two miles until being decapitated.

Laramie, Wyoming, October 7, 1998: A 21-year-old gay college student is lashed to a split-rail fence and pistol-whipped to the point where doctors are unable to perform surgery due to excessive cranial damage.

Greensburg, Pennsylvania, February 11, 2010: A 30-year-old mentally challenged woman is tortured for 36 hours before being stuffed in a garbage can and left for dead in a parking lot.

Although the heinousness alone of each of these crimes would presumably attract a large amount of media attention, it was the motivation behind these brutal attacks that brought about the most controversy. These victims were targeted and assaulted due to their perceived social status, making the attacks hate crimes.

Since the late 1980s, hate crimes have increasingly become the focus of public attention, shifting the lens of psychological and criminological research to address the causes and effects associated with this specific form of criminal behavior. Research on the topic has in turn fueled the advocacy of special laws protecting victims of hate crimes. Most recently, President Barack Obama signed into law the Matthew Shepard and James Byrd, Jr. Hate Crime Prevention Act of 2009 (18 U.S.C. § 249), increasing protection for lesbian, gay, bisexual and transgender individuals from attacks of hate and prejudice.

Past research has highlighted a variety of reasons for the occurrence of hate crimes, including resentment toward minority groups and a lack of governmental protection vis-à-vis civil rights (Craig, 2002). More personal contributing factors, such as in-group love, or feeling a strong sense of loyalty to one's group, as well as out-group hate, or having strong negative feelings toward those outside of one's group, have been proposed (Brewer, 1999). Conversely, some research has identified more symbolic motivations, such as religious beliefs (Swigonski, 2001) and the goal of conveying a message to a targeted group (Berk, 1990; Craig 2002). Taking all potential motivations into account while considering that rates at which the various types of hate crimes occur also differ, one might reasonably conclude that the experiences of each victim group may be vastly different.

The aim of this chapter is to discuss the unique experience of lesbian, gay, bisexual and transgender (LGBT) women who are victims of these crimes. By examining antifemale homosexual hate crimes within the context of hate crime in general, one is better able to appreciate the seriousness of these crimes and the effects that they have on both female and gay/lesbian groups as a whole. In order to do so, one must first understand the legal and societal perceptions of hate crimes in their most basic form.

WHAT IS A HATE CRIME?

A hate crime can be defined as "an offense in which the victim is targeted because of the actual or perceived race, color, religion, disability, sexual orientation, or national origin of that victim" (Sun, 2004, p. 597). Berk (1990) points out that because hate crimes are defined based on the determination of a perpetrator's motivation, the victim's actual status group is irrelevant in considering hate crimes. Rather, it is the perceived status group of the victim that motivates the offender's actions, and therefore caution should be used when considering crimes to be hate crimes. Because hate is a difficult concept to operationalize and objectively record, these offenses have been alternatively referred to as bias-motivated crimes, or crimes committed as an act of prejudice (Lawrence, 1999; McPhail, 2002). McPhail (2002) highlights the two distinct parts of a bias crime: the basic crime, such as an assault or vandalism, and the motivation that inspired it. Lawrence (1999) has described two models of bias crime: the discriminatory selection model and the animus model. In the former model, why an offender selected his or her victim on the basis of race or status is irrelevant; the fact that this selection was made is sufficient for deeming the incident a hate crime. The animus model is based on the offender's hatred of the victim's group membership, either actual or perceived. State statutes may use either or both of these models when criminalizing bias offenses (McPhail, 2002).

There is much variability in the way that hate crime incidents can occur. These types of incidents can involve more than one offense, victim, or offender (Cramer, 1999). Traditionally, the Federal Bureau of Investigation (FBI) has used 11 offense categories for crimes against persons and property in its collection of hate crime data: crimes against persons, which includes murder and nonnegligent manslaughter, forcible rape, robbery, aggravated assault, and intimidation, and crimes against property, which includes burglary, larceny or theft, motor vehicle theft, arson, simple assault, and destruction, damage, or vandalism of property. Those not fitting these categories are identified as crimes against society or other.

PREVALENCE OF HATE CRIMES IN THE UNITED STATES

In 2009, 2,034 law enforcement agencies reported 6,604 hate crime incidents involving 7,789 offenses (Federal Bureau of Investigation, 2010). Of these incidents, there were 6,598 single-bias incidents that involved 7,775 offenses, 8,322 victims, and 6,219 offenders: 3,816 (49.1%) were race-based offenses, 1,438 (18.5%) were sexual orientation–based offenses, 1,376 (17.7%) were religion-based offenses, 1,050 (13.5%) were ethnicity/national origin–based offenses, and 93 (1.2%) were disability-based offenses. Of the 7,789 offenses reported, 4,790 (61.5%) were crimes against persons, 3,653 (38.1%) were crimes against property, and 31 (.4%) were crimes against society. The most frequent type of offense across all bias motivations was destruction, damage, or vandalism (2,465, or 31.6%), with intimidation (2,158, or 27.7%) and simple assault (1,691, 21.7%) following closely. The most frequent location of offense across all bias motivations was the residence or home of the victim (2,070, or 31.3%), followed by highways, roads, alleys, or streets (1,135, or 17.2%) and schools or colleges (754, or 11.4%).

Specific differences can also be found within each bias motivation, with particular groups being more frequently victimized and the methods for doing so varying. According to he Federal Bureau of Investigation (2010), the majority of race-based offenses in 2009 were anti-Black (2,724, or 71.4%) and most frequently involved intimidation (935, or 34.3%) and destruction, damage, or vandalism (856, or 31.4%). The majority of sexual orientation–based hate crimes were against male homosexuals (798, or 55.6%) and most frequently involved simple assault (291, or 20.3%) and intimidation (170, or 11.8%). Of religion-based hate crimes in 2009, the majority (964, or 70%) were anti-Jewish and most commonly involved destruction, damage, or vandalism (671, or 69.6%). The majority of hate crimes based on ethnicity or national origin (654, or 62.3%) were anti-Hispanic in nature and usually involved intimidation (205, or 31.3%). Finally, disability-based hate crimes were reported to be most frequently motivated by an anti–mental disability bias (72, or 74.2%) and most commonly involved destruction, damage, or vandalism (17, or 23.6%) and simple assault (17, or 23.6%).

HATE CRIME LEGISLATION

Although the 1964 Federal Civil Rights Law (18 U.S.C. § 245) was established to prosecute anyone who "willingly injures, intimidates or interferes with another person, or attempts to do so, by force because of the other person's race, color, religion or national origin," this law failed to recognize a number of marginalized groups. Additionally, this law only applied to those acts in which the perpetrator was attempting to prevent the victim from engaging in any of five types of federally protected activities: being in a public place or facility, applying for a job, voting, attending school, or serving as a juror.

An increased awareness of the type and nature of these hate crimes or bias-motivated crimes has resulted in a string of legislative action by the U.S. government starting in the early 1990s. On April 23, 1990, Congress passed the Hate Crime Statistics Act, which required the attorney general to collect data "about crimes that manifest evidence of prejudice based on race, religion, sexual orientation, or ethnicity" (Hate Crime Statistics Act, 1990). The FBI was put in charge of developing the procedures for implementing the collection and management of hate crime data and consequently assigned the tasks to the Uniform Crime Reporting (UCR) Program. Through the cooperation and assistance of many local and state law enforcement agencies, hate crime data collection became possible.

The UCR Program's first publication, *Hate Crime Statistics, 1990: A Resource Book* (1993), was a compilation of hate crime data from 11 states that were willing to offer their 1990 data as a prototype. The FBI worked closely with agencies familiar with investigating hate crimes and collecting related information so that it could develop and implement a more uniform method of data collection on a nationwide scale. *Hate Crime Statistics, 1992,* presented the first published data reported by law enforcement agencies across the country that participated in the UCR Hate Crime Statistics Program. Since this time, the Hate Crime Statistics Act has been amended on several occasions to increase protection for particular groups.

In September 1994, lawmakers amended the Hate Crime Statistics Act to include bias against persons with disabilities. Because persons with disabilities can be considered an especially vulnerable minority group (McMahon, West, Lewis, Armstrong, & Conway, 2004) and disability has been shown to be a basis of discrimination (Fine & Asch, 1988), the government passed the Violent Crime Control and Law Enforcement Act of 1994 (28 U.S.C. § 994). Furthermore, the act increased the penalties for all hate-based crimes involving the protected groups of "race, color, religion, national origin, ethnicity, gender, disability, or sexual orientation" (Cogan, 2002, p. 175). It was not until January 1, 1997, however, that the FBI started gathering data for the additional bias types.

Other important legislative actions include the passing of the Hate Crimes Sentencing Enhancement Act of 1994, a controversial act that enforces increased punishment for hate crime offenders, and the Church Arson Prevention Act of 1996 (H.R. 3525, 104th Congress), which mandates that the collection of hate crime data become a permanent part of the UCR Program (Federal Bureau of Investigation, 2010).

Most recently, Congress further amended the Hate Crime Statistics Act by passing the Matthew Shepard and James Byrd, Jr. Hate Crime Prevention Act of 2009 (18 U.S.C. § 534). The amendment extends the collection of data to crimes motivated by bias against a particular gender and gender identity as well as for crimes committed by and crimes directed against juveniles. The FBI is currently making plans to implement changes to collect these data (Federal Bureau of Investigation, 2010).

REACTIONS TO HATE CRIME LEGISLATION

As can be evidenced by the trend in legislative action, there is an array of arguments in support of hate crime–specific legislation. Among these arguments is the idea that hate crimes, unlike non–hate crimes, affect not only the individual victim but also the whole group to which the victim belongs (Cogan, 2002; Iganski, 2001). To put this into perspective, if an individual is targeted for an assault due to her or his actual or perceived sexual orientation, it is quite possible that the entire LGBT community may experience the repercussions of the attack. This violation of basic human rights based on sexual preference may result in a pervasive and community-wide experience of negative emotions such as fear and depression. Furthermore, Craig (1999) found that responses of other in-group members to hate crimes were more likely to include retaliation even when the emotions reported by in-group and out-group members were similar. These results imply that hate crimes are more likely than non–hate crimes to foster future violence (Craig, 1999). As was evidenced in the riots that occurred in Los Angeles at the close of the trial of White police officers who had beaten an African American man, Rodney King, the impact of hate crimes reaches far past the effect on an individual victim.

Franklin (2002) points out that hate crime legislation has helped to better protect those who have historically been victimized by shedding light on the severity and unique nature of bias-motivated crimes. Despite an increase in the awareness and recording of hate crimes, the effectiveness of hate crime legislation has fallen under scrutiny. Critics of hate crime legislation highlight the various pitfalls involved with the actual justification and implementation of these new laws: it is often incredibly difficult to determine the motivation of an act, especially when the offender is unknown (Cogan, 2002; Franklin, 2002); there is a large degree of variability in the way hate crimes are categorized across agencies (Franklin, 2002); and there are inherent weaknesses in the argument that hate crimes more negatively impact victims than non–hate-motivated crimes

(Iganski, 2001). Perhaps the most important criticism is presented by Bakken (2002), who emphasizes the limited availability and reliability of hate crime statistics. While hate crime statistics are a mandated portion of UCR data, this data is compiled from the voluntary participation of law enforcement agencies around the country. Because it has also been suggested that hate crimes are less likely to be reported (Herek, Cogan, & Gillis, 2002), this issue is further emphasized.

While it is difficult to provide large-scale empirical support for a number of arguments for and against hate crime legislation, it is important to explore the societal perceptions of such crimes and the possible factors that may affect an individual's reactions to these laws. Researchers have suggested many factors that might influence someone's support of or opposition to hate crime legislation. At the most basic level, an individual's own demographics or characteristics may influence her or his perception of hate crimes. These characteristics include not only demographic factors, such as one's race, gender, age, and education level, but also beliefs and attitudes, such as social and economic liberalism as well as beliefs regarding punishment (Craig & Waldo, 1996; Quist & Wiegend, 2002) and attitudes toward homosexuality (Quist & Wiegand, 2002; Johnson & Byers, 2003). For example, Craig and Waldo (1996) found that participants of color and females were more likely than White or male participants to identify a hate crime. In regard to issues affecting jury sentencing and decision making, Haegerich and Bottoms (2000) found that when empathy toward the defendant was induced in jurors, female jurors were more likely than male jurors to believe the defendant and find him or her guilty less often. Other factors may include the presence of verbal aggression in an offense and an individual's perceptions of hate crime characteristics, such as prevalence and the influence of fear that is instilled by these crimes (Quist & Wiegand, 2002). It is possible that both individuals who believe hate crime victims to be more negatively impacted than their non–hate crime counterparts and those who support hate crime legislation are more likely to display higher levels of empathy for the hate crime victims than for victims of crimes without an apparent bias motivation.

Independent of societal perceptions, it is clear that hate crime victim experiences may differ due to a number of interacting factors. In order to better understand the significance of hate crimes for gay and lesbian women, it is first important to understand the effect that such crimes have on the LGBT community in general.

SEXUAL ORIENTATION HATE CRIMES

In addition to government organizations tracking hate crimes, the National Coalition of Anti-Violence Programs (National Coalition of Anti-Violence Programs, 1997) collects data on antigay hate crimes from local and state antiviolence programs. This organization uses a particular definition for documenting a sexual orientation hate crime: "one in which there are sufficient objective facts to lead a reasonable person to conclude that the offender's bias against lesbian, gay, bisexual, transgender, or HIV-Positive people" (National Coalition of Anti-Violence Programs, 1997, p. 2).

According to the Federal Bureau of Investigation (2010), the breakdown of sexual orientation hate crimes by victim type in 2009 was as follows: of the 1,482 victims, 55.1% were victims because of an offender's anti–male homosexual bias, 26.4% were victims because of an antihomosexual bias, 15.3% were victims because of an anti–female homosexual bias, 1.8% were victims because of an antibisexual bias, and 1.4% were victims because of an antiheterosexual bias.

Dunbar (2006) and Willis (2004) conclude that sexual orientation hate crimes may in fact systematically differ from other types of hate crimes in severity of violence. Based on research, more violent and brutal forms of aggression were found in sexual orientation–motivated hate crimes. Findings concluded that "assault, sexual assault, sexual harassment/attempted assault and stalking" were more strongly associated with hate crimes based on sexual orientation, while all other hate crime motivations were found to be more strongly associated with "assault with a deadly weapon, being a target of either printed or verbal hate speech, and hate graffiti activity" (Dunbar, 2006, p. 330). Furthermore, several researchers have demonstrated that due to the nature of the offenses most frequently found in sexual orientation hate crimes, victims are less likely to report the offense than are victims of other hate crimes (Bernstein & Kostelac, 2002; Dunbar, 2006; Herek et al., 2002; Peel, 1999). These findings begin to highlight potential differences in the experiences of hate crime victims and the attitudes behind each bias crime. It is therefore important to understand these unique differences in potential perpetrator attitudes in sexual orientation hate crimes as well as the experiences of and impacts on the mental health of LGBT individuals and LGBT women as compared to other hate crime victims.

WHERE AND HOW SEXUAL ORIENTATION DISCRIMINATION AND HATE CRIMES OCCUR

Just as the basis for attitudes behind sexual orientation–based hate crimes can be diverse, so too can the locations in which such acts occur. Herek (2000) posits that sexual prejudice can stem from bad interactions with LGBT individuals generalized to the whole LGBT community, fear in relation to homosexuality, the influence of other in-group members, or beliefs that homosexuality goes against one's values and morals. These attitudes may be held by a variety of individuals and cannot therefore be isolated to one type of person or to one type of location. Poll data indicated that more than half of the adults in the United States held negative attitudes toward lesbians and gay men and always felt that homosexual behavior was wrong (Yang, 1997). In the same poll, a majority opposed legalizing same-sex marriage and did not believe that lesbians and gay men should be allowed to adopt children (Yang, 1997). Because these prejudicial attitudes toward LGBT individuals are widely held, potential perpetrators may be found anywhere. As such, individuals may be targeted in any or all aspects of their lives, whether it be by a family member at home, a peer at school, a colleague at work, or even strangers or society as a whole.

According to the FBI Uniform Crime Reports, the majority of hate crimes with a sexual orientation bias motivation in 2009 occurred in a residence, followed by a highway, road, alley, or street; other or unknown; and a school or college (Federal Bureau of Investigation, 2010). In reviewing the literature on where LGBT individuals have experienced hate crimes, Cheng (2004) points out that the location of these crimes runs the gamut from schools to homes, courtrooms, prisons, and media outlets, among others. Herek et al. (2002) found that compared to nonbias person crimes, bias person crimes occurred more often in public places and were more likely to involve multiple perpetrators who were strangers to the victim. However, in their sample, victims of sexual orientation hate crimes reported being victimized at home, at school, in the workplace, and by friends and family members (Herek et al., 2002). In a prior study, Herek, Gillis, Cogan, and Glunt (1997) found that the majority of female victims of sexual orientation–based hate crimes were attacked by someone they knew, while the majority of male victims were attacked by strangers. Additionally, a majority of the female victims were attacked in a private setting such as their home, while a majority of the male victims were attacked in a public setting (Herek et al., 1997). Thus, lesbians and bisexual women may be more likely to be victimized in various aspects of their daily lives, as the majority of one's time is spent at home, school, or work where they are at least acquainted with those surrounding them.

Family/Home

Discrimination based on one's sexual orientation as well as sexual orientation–based hate crimes may be experienced at one's home and may begin to occur as early as adolescence. For many LGBT individuals, coming out is a significant part of their lives and is thus accompanied by high levels of stress regarding how others, especially family members, are going to react and whether or not they will accept the LGBT individual. In a survey by Yang (1997), a majority of adult respondents across the United States stated that they would not be accepting if their child admitting to being homosexual. Furthermore, these respondents also stated that they would be upset or that they would feel that the relationship between themselves and their child would subsequently be negatively affected (Yang, 1997). Similarly, in a study examining parental response to finding out that their adolescent was homosexual, Saltzburg (2004) found that the parents reported having felt overwhelmed by the information and that they no longer knew how to parent their child. They also reported experiencing feelings of sadness and deep loss, subsequently emotionally detaching from their teenage child (Saltzburg, 2004). Participants in a study who were asked to share their sexual orientation–based hate crime experiences reported having been victimized by a family member such as a parent or sibling; for example, one participant reported having been beaten by her mother after she had gotten drunk in response to finding out that her daughter was a lesbian (Herek et al., 2002). Thus, teens as well as young adults may experience discrimination and potentially hate crimes in the home based on their sexual orientation.

Sexual minorities may also experience hate crimes at their home by perpetrators who may be strangers, neighbors, or other acquaintances and know where the individual lives. In a study examining the various aspects of sexual orientation–based hate crimes, Herek et al. (2002) found that LGBT individuals are targeted at home. Specifically, participants reported having had their cars, houses, or other property vandalized, stolen, or damaged or having been targets of sexual orientation slurs and other verbal harassment at their residence. These hate crimes were reportedly perpetrated by neighbors who were aware of their sexual orientation or as a result of having participated in a public event or act that identified them as homosexual (Herek et al., 2002). This was an extension of a previous study conducted by Herek et al. (1997), results of which indicated that especially for women, sexual orientation–based hate crimes often occurred in the victims' home or the perpetrator's home by someone the victim knew. This is likely to result in LGBT individuals having difficulty finding a safe haven where they can be free of discrimination and hate crime victimization.

Peers/School

Adolescents and young adults in school may find themselves being targeted due to their sexual orientation by their peers or intimate partners. Herek et al. (2002) found that respondents recalled being targets of antigay harassment in middle and secondary school. Furthermore, participants reported having been victims of sexual orientation–based hate crimes on their college campuses as well (Herek et al., 2002). In a study of high school students, sexual minority adolescents were more likely than their heterosexual counterparts to report having been victims of bullying and sexual harassment (Williams, Connolly, Pepler, & Craig, 2005). LGBT individuals may also be victimized by their intimate partners or ex-partners. Intimate partner violence can be found in heterosexual as well as homosexual relationships, although there are differences in the ways in which the violence is manifested (Freedner, Freed, Yang, & Austin, 2002). Freedner et al. (2002) found that in a community survey of adolescents, bisexual males were more likely to have experienced any type of abuse by an intimate partner than were heterosexual individuals, and bisexual individuals were more likely to report having been threatened with outing by an intimate partner than were lesbians and gay men. Furthermore, bisexual females were more likely than any other group to have been sexually abused by an intimate partner (Freedner et al., 2002). In Herek et al.'s (2002) sample, female participants reported having been sexually abused by ex-husbands or ex-boyfriends who had felt rejected by them or by male friends who would not believe that the woman was a lesbian. LGBT individuals therefore may be victimized by their peers at school or within their relationships.

Some research has focused on exploring the reasons behind such occurrences in schools by looking at attitudes held by adolescents and young adults regarding sexual minorities. High school–aged heterosexual students were surveyed about their attitudes toward sexual minorities and the rights of these individuals (Horn, Szalacha, & Drill, 2008). While respondents reported feeling that their LGBT peers have the right to be and feel safe in school, they still held negative attitudes toward sexual minorities and reported justifications for holding such beliefs (Horn et al., 2008). This may mean that while adolescents can theoretically acknowledge the rights of their LGBT peers, they may be unaware of times in which they may be discriminating against or victimizing LGBT individuals and thus infringing on their rights to safety. The reasons they use to justify their attitudes may also be utilized in justifying any antigay behavior. Franklin (2002) administered an anonymous survey to noncriminal young adults and found that 1 in 10 admitted to having physically abused or threatened a presumed homosexual, and roughly 1 in 4 admitted to verbally abusing a presumed homosexual. Four motivational themes emerged from this data: antigay ideology, perceived self-defense, thrill seeking, and peer dynamics (Franklin, 2002). This suggests that LGBT individuals may be targeted for a variety of reasons, perhaps not just hate alone. Similarly, Miller (2001) examined students' perception of victims of hate crimes and found that White males who were not criminal justice students were less likely than their female counterparts to label individuals as hate crime victims for all four hate crime scenarios with Jewish, African American, female, and sexual minority victims. Furthermore, criminal justice male students were less likely than their female counterparts to classify females and sexual minorities as hate crime victims (Miller, 2001). These findings may begin to suggest why sexual minorities and particularly female sexual minorities experience hate crimes in a variety of different locations and in potentially unique ways.

Colleagues/Work

Discrimination against sexual minorities in the workplace can take on many forms. For example, LGBT individuals may be discriminated against while looking for jobs through the hiring process. Horvath and Ryan (2003) found that negative attitudes toward sexual minorities correlated with beliefs about employing them and subsequently hiring discrimination. Many of these beliefs were rooted in traditional gender roles and whether or not employers thought that an LGBT individual would be able to perform the job as a result of nonconforming (Horvath & Ryan, 2003). Yang (1997) found that a majority of adults polled in the United States did not support the hiring of lesbians and gay men in certain professions such as in health care and the clergy. Thus, preconceived notions and negative attitudes toward the LGBT community may already work against a sexual minority individual when applying for jobs.

Once hired, LGBT individuals may find themselves in the predicament of whether or not to come out to coworkers, or if they already have they may find themselves being targeted due to their sexuality. Waldo (1999) found that outness was positively correlated with direct heterosexism in the workplace; therefore, many LGBT individuals find themselves experiencing discrimination due to their sexual orientation if they are out at work. Ragins and Cornwell (2001) also found that outness was related to discrimination and that workplaces with predominantly heterosexual environments and without supportive policies and protective legislation were more likely to have discrimination occurring within their walls.

Society

LGBT individuals may also feel victimized by society as a whole in a variety of different ways and locations. For example, Yang (1997) found in an opinion poll that a majority of adults across the United States are opposed to gay marriage or adoption. Because such attitudes are widespread and widely held, LGBT individuals have the potential to be discriminated against anywhere. Furthermore, as a result of these attitudes, most states do not allow gay marriage, and discrimination is thus felt at a societal level. Additionally, discrimination and hate crimes against sexual minorities may occur within law enforcement agencies as well as through their work with the public. For example, Bernstein and Kostelac (2002) asked police officers their opinions regarding LGBT individuals in law enforcement agencies as well as in the community. Fifteen percent of these officers felt that LGBT police officers undermined their abilities to be good role models for the community, and 25% felt that hiring LGBT police officers would negatively affect the morale at work (Bernstein & Kostelac, 2002). Between 10% and 20% admitted to some form of antigay behavior, only 60% said that they treat homosexual and heterosexual community members similarly, and only 72% felt that calls from homosexual individuals were taken as seriously as and were dealt with similarly to calls made by heterosexual individuals (Bernstein & Kostelac, 2002). LGBT individuals therefore may feel when interacting with society and specifically law enforcement agencies that they are likely to experience further discrimination.

Subsequently, perceptions of police attitudes toward homosexual individuals may lead to underreporting of sexual orientation–based hate crimes. Peel (1999) did in fact find that perceptions of police attitudes, specifically that police generally hold negative antigay attitudes and would therefore not treat the crime as seriously, were reasons behind nonreporting. Herek et al. (2002) found that victims of bias crimes were less likely than victims of nonbias crimes to report the incident and furthermore that while bisexual men were the least likely to report bias crimes (with bisexual women and lesbians next likely to report), lesbians had the biggest difference in reporting between nonbias- and bias-related crimes. Dunbar (2006) also found that reporting was related to the severity of the bias crime in that more violent aggression led to underreporting. Therefore, LGBT individuals may experience discrimination and hate crimes at a societal level, thus affecting the way they live, the choices they make following victimization, and their ability to feel a sense of justice, closure, and safety after the crime.

WOMEN'S UNIQUE EXPERIENCES

Lesbian and bisexual women may experience more workplace discrimination than gay and bisexual men, as was found in a study conducted by Herek et al. (2002). Lesbian and bisexual women reported more workplace hate crime victimization, especially in traditional male settings such as law enforcement agencies (Herek et al., 2002). For example, Bernstein and Kostelac (2002) found that more police officers thought that compared to nonlesbians, lesbians could not be as effective as police officers, but those same officers polled rated higher the potential for gay males to be effective police officers compared to nongay males. Furthermore, lesbians and bisexual females face the possibility of being targeted due to their gender as well as their sexual orientation. In a study examining prosecutors' perspectives on gender-bias crimes in Texas, McPhail and DiNitto (2005) found that only a quarter of the men and half the women could see violence against women as a hate crime, and a majority did not know that gender had been included in the Texas legislation on hate crimes. This may suggest that violence against women is not perceived to be as serious as that against other protected groups and may therefore occur more frequently without any resultant action against the perpetrator. Crow, Fok, and Hartman (1998) examined LGBT individuals' experiences with workplace discrimination and found that Black homosexuals were most likely to be victimized, followed by White female homosexuals and then White male homosexuals. This too suggests possible combinations of race, gender, and sexual orientation discrimination leading lesbians and female bisexuals, and especially those who are also racial minorities, to possibly experience more discrimination than their male counterparts.

Effects of Sexual Orientation Discrimination and Hate Crimes

The legislation associated with hate crimes has increased the penalties for all crimes committed against protected groups, implying that hate- or bias-motivated crimes are considered more severe than non–hate crimes or non–bias crimes. Research indeed has shown that hate crimes tend to have a greater impact on victims than do non–hate crimes (Herek et al., 2002; McDevitt, Balboni, Garcia, & Gu, 2000). For example, Herek et al. (2002) found that LGBT individuals who were victims of bias crimes within the previous five years reported greater levels of psychological distress than their non–bias crime victim counterparts. Furthermore, this psychological distress tended to be longer lasting and more severe for the victims of bias crimes than for victims of non–bias crimes (Herek et al., 2002). Similar results were found in a study examining the differences in impact for bias crime victims and non–bias crime victims; levels of depression, fear of one's safety, nervousness, and intrusive thoughts were all significantly higher for victims of bias crimes than victims of non–bias crimes (McDevitt et al., 2000). McDevitt et al. (2000) also reported that these effects were experienced by bias crime victims over longer periods of time than victims of similar non–bias crimes. Barnes and Ephross (1994) found that the most reported emotional responses to victimization included fear, sadness, and anger.

Effects on LGBT Victims

While research has reported differences between the effects of hate crimes and non–hate crimes, there has also been research examining the unique experiences of victims of LGBT discrimination and hate crimes. Discrimination against LGBT individuals, especially if experienced continually, has been found to have detrimental impacts on the targeted individual's mental health and daily functioning. Ueno (2005) found that the impacts of sexual orientation discrimination can be seen as early as adolescence; the sexual minority teens in his study reported greater levels of psychological distress than their heterosexual counterparts. Research has also found that sexual minority youths have higher levels of substance use than heterosexual teens (Corliss et al., 2010; Marshall et al., 2008). For LGBT adolescents, victimization and substance use, victimization and depression/suicidal thoughts, and substance use and depression/suicidal thoughts all had higher correlations than for their heterosexual counterparts (Poteat, Aragon, Espelage, & Koenig, 2009). Sexual orientation discrimination can also occur when these individuals are older and in the workplace on a daily basis. Chung (1995) highlighted the effects that can be felt by LGBT individuals even before they have a job when they are making career decisions, in that they think about ways in which they may be victimized in different job markets and how they may subsequently feel after experiencing such discrimination. Specifically, "He or she may experience isolation, avoidance, negative attitudes, harassment, or even physical assault in the workplace because of people's homophobia, negative stereotypes, and societal stigmas" (Chung 1995, p. 183). Research has also found that heterosexism and perceived discrimination against LGBT individuals in the workplace are associated with psychological distress (Waldo, 1999) and job dissatisfaction (Day & Schoenrade, 1997; Waldo, 1999). Furthermore, perceived discrimination in the workplace has also been found to be associated with fewer promotions and with negative work attitudes (Ragins & Cornwell, 2001).

Just as LGBT victims of discrimination may experience unique effects on their functioning and mental health, so too may LGBT hate crime victims. For instance, Dunbar (2006) examined the differences in the impact of hate crimes between victims in different protected groups and found that LGBT hate crime victims reported greater impact on their daily functioning than did victims of religious hate crimes, which was significant, and greater, but not significantly different, effects than victims of racial/ethnic hate crimes. Williams et al. (2005) reported their results that sexual minority adolescents' peer victimization was associated with psychological symptoms such as depression and also with more externalizing behaviors. Posttraumatic stress disorder (PTSD) symptoms have also been found in LGBT victims of hate crimes (Cheng, 2004; Herek et al., 1997; Herek, Gillis, & Cogan, 1999) along with increased levels of anger, depression, and anxiety (Herek et al., 1997; Herek et al., 1999). Furthermore, LGBT victims of hate crimes are more likely to report less belief in the benevolence of people (Herek et al., 1997) as well as to be more likely to have crime-related fears and beliefs, a lower sense of mastery, and increased blame on sexual prejudice for their personal setbacks (Herek et al., 1999). Thus, a variety of negative emotional reactions and behavioral responses are experienced by LGBT individuals as a result of being targeted and victimized on the basis of hate.

Effects on Lesbian and Bisexual Female Victims

Little research has been conducted to examine the unique experiences of LGBT women as victims of hate crimes and the potential differences in the impact of LGBT hate crimes between male and female victims. Although Szymanski (2005) only examined LGBT women, it is worth noting that internalized heterosexism, recent sexist events, recent sexual orientation–based hate crime victimization, and the interaction of the latter two were all found to be significant predictors of psychological distress. Poteat et al. (2009) found that adolescent sexual minority females were more likely to report depression/suicidal thoughts than adolescent sexual minority males. While Corliss et al. (2010) found that sexually minority adolescents reported greater substance use than heterosexual adolescents and also found that the effect size was greater for females. Similarly, research has also shown that a significant correlation between adolescent sexual orientation and substance abuse was greatest for bisexual females (Marshal et al., 2008). As for intimate partner violence, lesbians have reported greater fear regarding their safety than any other sexual minority group (Freedner et al., 2002).

In conjunction with LGBT discrimination and hate crime victimization, LGBT women may also be targeted based on other aspects or characteristics of themselves and thus may be targeted more often and affected more by such experiences. Racial minority LGBT women have reported higher levels of depression and suicidal thoughts than White LGBT women, although this difference was not significant (Poteat et al., 2009). LGBT women may also be targeted based not only on their sexual orientation but also on their gender, adding to the effects of discrimination and hate crime victimization. Women in the workplace, for example, experience gender discrimination in the form of gender harassment and sexual harassment or unwanted sexual attention, which may lead to decreased job satisfaction and life satisfaction as well as increased mental health issues and PTSD symptoms (Schneider, Swan, & Fitzgerald, 1997). LGBT women and LGBT racial minorities therefore may be at a greater risk of victimization and may consequently be affected even more than LGBT White individuals and LGBT men.

CONCLUSION

While research has begun to look at various aspects of hate crimes such as what constitutes a hate crime, its associated legislation, the effects of hate crime victimization and societal attitudes regarding all of these facets (Barnes & Ephross, 1994; Cogan, 2002; Iganski, 2001; McDevitt et al., 2000; Yang, 1997), more research is still needed. Specifically, while the bases of sexual orientation–based hate crimes are different than other bias crimes, it may also follow that the effects of such victimization differ. Furthermore, research has begun to show that belonging to more than one minority group may result in increased victimization, the additive nature of which may result in more adverse effects on these individuals' mental health and daily functioning. As such, future research should focus on the experiences of members belonging to more than one minority group such as LGBT women or Black LGBT women, as these individuals may be more susceptible to victimization and the consequences of being targeted.

REFERENCES

Association of State Uniform Crime Reporting Programs (U.S.), Northeastern University (Boston, Mass.), Center for Applied Social Research (U.S.), & Federal Bureau of Investigation (1993). *Hate crime statistics, 1990: A resource book.* Darby, PA: DIANE Publishing.

Bakken, T. (2002). The effects of hate crime legislation: Unproven benefits and unintended consequences. *International Journal of Discrimination and the Law, 5,* 231–246.

Barnes, A., & Ephross, P. (1994). The impact of hate violence on victims: Emotional and behavioral responses to attacks. *Social Work, 39,* 247–251.

Berk, R. (1990). Thinking about hate-motivated crimes. *Journal of Interpersonal Violence, 5,* 334–349.

Bernstein, M., & Kostelac, C. (2002). Lavender and blue: Attitudes about homosexuality and behavior toward lesbians and gay men among police officers. *Journal of Contemporary Criminal Justice, 18,* 302–328.

Brewer, M. B. (1999). The psychology of prejudice: Ingroup love or outgroup hate? *Journal of Social Issues, 55,* 429–444.

Cheng, Z. (2004). Hate crimes, post-traumatic stress disorder and implications for counseling lesbians and gay men. *Journal of Applied Rehabilitation Couseling, 35,* 8–16.

Chung, Y. B. (1995). Career decision making of lesbian, gay, and bisexual individuals. *Career Development Quarterly, 44,* 178–190.

Cogan, J. C. (2002). Hate crimes as a crime category worthy of policy attention. *American Behavioral Scientist, 46,* 173–185.

Corliss, H. L., Rosario, M., Wypij, D., Wylie, S. A., Frazier, A. L., & Austin, S. B. (2010). Sexual orientation and drug use in a longitudinal cohort study of U.S. adolescents. *Addictive Behaviors, 35,* 517–521.

Craig, K. M. (1999). Retaliation, fear, or rage: An investigation of African-American and White reactions to racist hate crimes. *Journal of Interpersonal Violence, 14,* 138–151.

Craig, K. M. (2002). Examining hate-motivated aggression: A review of the social psychological literature on hate crimes as a distinct form of aggression. *Aggression and Violent Behavior, 7,* 85–101.

Craig, K. M., & Waldo, C. R. (1996). "So, what's a hate crime anyway?" Young adults' perceptions of hate crimes, victims, and perpetrators. *Law and Human Behavior, 20,* 113–129.

Cramer, E. P. (1999). Hate crime laws and sexual orientation. *Journal of Sociology and Social Welfare, 26,* 5–24.

Crow, S. M., Fok, L. Y., & Hartman, S. J. (1998). Who is at greatest risk of work-related discrimination—Women, blacks, or homosexuals? *Employee Responsibilities and Rights Journal, 11,* 15–26.

Day, N. E., & Schoenrade, P. (1997). Staying in the closet versus coming out: Relationships between communication about sexual orientation and work attitudes. *Personnel Psychology, 50,* 147–163.

Dunbar, E. (2006). Race, gender, and sexual orientation in hate crime victimization: Identity politics or identity risk? *Violence and Victims, 21,* 323–337.

Federal Bureau of Investigation (2010, October). *Hate Crime Statistics, 2009.* Washington, DC: U.S. Department of Justice, Federal Bureau of Investigation.

Federal Civil Rights Law, 18 U.S.C. §245 (1964).

Fine, M. & Asch, A. (1988). Disability beyond stigma: Social interaction, discrimination, and activism. *Journal of Social Issues, 44,* 3–21.

Franklin, K. (2002). Good intentions: The enforcement of hate crime penalty-enhancement statutes. *American Behavioral Scientist, 46,* 154–172.

Freedner, N., Freed, L. H., Yang, Y. W., & Austin, S. B. (2002). Dating violence among gay, lesbian, and bisexual adolescents: Results from a community survey. *Journal of Adolescent Health, 31,* 469 474.

Haegerich, T., & Bottoms, B. L. (2000). Empathy and jurors' decisions in patricide trials involving child sexual assault allegations. *Law and Human Behavior, 24,* 421–448.

Hate Crime Sentencing Enhancement Act, 28 U.S.C. §994 (1994).

Hate Crime Statistics Act, 28 U.S.C. §534 (1990).

Herek, G. M. (2000). The psychology of sexual prejudice. *Current Directions in Psychological Science, 9,* 19–22.

Herek, G. M., Cogan, J. C., & Gillis, R. J. (2002). Victim experiences in hate crime based on sexual orientation. *Journal of Social Issues, 58,* 319–339.

Herek, G. M., Gillis, R. J., & Cogan, J. C. (1999). Psychological sequelae of hate-crime victimization among lesbian, gay, and bisexual adults. *Journal of Consulting and Clinical Psychology, 67,* 945–951.

Herek, G. M., Gillis, R. J., Cogan, J. C., & Glunt, E. K. (1997). Hate crime victimization among lesbian, gay, and bisexual adults: Prevalence, psychological correlates, and methodological issues. *Journal of Interpersonal Violence, 12,* 195–215.

Horn, S. S., Szalacha, L. A., Drill, K. (2008). Schooling, sexuality, and rights: An investigation of heterosexual students' social cognition regarding sexual orientation and the rights of gay and lesbian peers in school. *Journal of Social Issues, 64,* 791–813.

Horvath, M., & Ryan, A. M. (2003). Antecedents and potential moderators of the relationship between attitudes and hiring discrimination on the basis of sexual orientation. *Sex Roles, 48,* 115–130.

H.R. 3525, 104th Congress, Church Arson Prevention Act of 1996. (1996). In GovTrack. us [Database of federal legislation]. Retrieved on November 7, 2010, from http://www.govtrack.us/congress/bill.xpd?bill=h104-3525&tab=summary.

Iganski, P. (2001). Hate crimes hurt more. *American Behavioral Scientist, 45,* 626–638.

Johnson, S. D., & Byers, B. D. (2003). Attitudes toward hate crime laws. *Journal of Criminal Justice, 31,* 227–235.

Lawrence, F. M. (1999). *Punishing hate bias crimes under American law.* Cambridge: Harvard University Press.

Marshall, M. P., Friedman, M. S., Stall, R., King, K. M., Miles, J., Gold, M. A., Bukstein, O. G., & Morse, J. Q. (2008). Sexual orientation and adolescent substance use: A meta-analysis and methodological review. *Addiction, 103,* 546–556.

Matthew Shepard and James Byrd, Jr. Hate Crime Prevention Act, 18 U.S.C. §249 (2009).
McDevitt, J., Balboni, J., Garcia, L., & Gu, J. (2000). Consequences for victims: A comparison of bias– and non-bias–motivated assaults. *American Behavioral Scientist, 45,* 697–713.
McMahon, B. T., West, S. L., Lewis, A. N., Armstrong, A. J., & Conway, J. P. (2004). Hate crimes and disability in America. *Rehabilitation Counseling Bulletin, 47,* 66–75.
McPhail, B. A. (2002). Gender-bias hate crimes: A review. *Trauma, Violence, and Abuse, 3,* 125–143.
McPhail, B. A., & DiNitto, D. M. (2005). Prosecutorial perspectives on gender-bias hate crimes. *Violence Against Women, 11,* 1162–1185.
Miller, A. J. (2001). Student perceptions of hate crimes. *American Journal of Criminal Justice, 25,* 293–307.
National Coalition of Anti-Violence Programs (1997). Anti-GLBTH incidents in 1997. Retrieved on November 7, 2010, from www.lambda.org/1997_national_rpt.pdf.
Peel, F. (1999). Violence against lesbians and gay men: Decision-making in reporting and not reporting crime. *Feminism & Psychology, 9,* 161–167.
Poteat, V. P., Aragon, S. R., Espelage, D. L., & Koenig, B. W. (2009). Psychosocial concerns of sexual minority youth: Complexity and caution in group differences. *Journal of Consulting and Clinical Psychology, 77,* 196–201.
Quist, R. M., & Wiegand, D. M. (2002). Attributions of hate: The media's causal attributions of a homophobic murder. *American Behavioral Scientist, 46,* 93–107.
Ragins, B. R., & Cornwell, J. M. (2001). Pink triangles: Antecedents and consequences of perceived workplace discrimination against gay and lesbian employees. *Journal of Applied Psychology, 86,* 1244–1261.
Saltzburg, S. (2004). Learning that an adolescent child is gay or lesbian: The parent experience. *Social Work, 49,* 109–118.
Schneider, K. T., Swann, S., & Fitzgerald, L. F. (1997) Job-related and psychological effects of sexual harassment in the workplace: Empirical evidence from two organizations. *Journal of Applied Psychology, 82,* 401–415.
Sun, K. (2004). The legal definition of hate crime and the hate offender's distorted cognitions. *Issues in Mental Health Nursing, 27,* 597–604.
Swigonski, M. E. (2001). Human rights, hate crimes, and Hebrew-Christian scripture. *Journal of Gay & Lesbian Social Services: Issues in Practice, Policy & Research, 13,* 33–45.
Szymanski, D. M. (2005). Heterosexism and sexism as correlates of psychological distress in lesbians. *Journal of Counseling & Development, 83,* 355–360.
Ueno, K. (2005). Sexual orientation and psychological distress in adolescence: Examining interpersonal stressors and social support processes. *Social Psychology Quarterly, 68,* 258–277.
Violent Crime Control and Law Enforcement Act, 28 U.S.C. §994 (1994).
Waldo, C. R. (1999). Working in a majority context: A structural model of heterosexism as minority stress in the workplace. *Journal of Counseling Psychology, 46,* 218–232.
Williams, T., Connolly, J., Pepler, D., & Craig, W. (2005). Peer victimization, social support, and psychosocial adjustment of sexual minority adolescents. *Journal of Youth and Adolescence, 34,* 471–482.
Willis, D. G. (2004). Hate crimes against gay males: An overview. *Issues in Mental Health Nursing, 25,* 115–132.
Yang, A. S. (1997). The polls-trends: Attitudes toward homosexuality. *Public Opinion Quarterly, 61,* 477–507.

Chapter 8

Abuse in Adulthood

William E. Schweinle

MENTAL HEALTH CONSEQUENCES AND CORRELATES OF PARTNER ABUSE

In the United States roughly 1.5 million women are physically or sexually abused by their male partner each year (Centers for Disease Control and Prevention, 2003). The mental health consequences for these women has been the subject of substantial scientific investigation during the past 30 years (for a summary, see Warshaw, Brashler, & Gil, 2009), though more research into the psychological sequelae of abuse is certainly warranted. Greater understanding of women's abuse-precipitated psychological harm will help inform the treatment of abused women, whose psychological injuries can be more difficult to identify and can often take longer to heal than physical ones (see Davidson & van der Kolk, 1996).

On the one hand, the majority of women victims of intimate partner violence do not have long-term mental health issues (Briere, Woo, McRae, Foltz, & Sitzman, 1997; Goodman, Dutton, & Harris, 1997). On the other hand, abused women usually do experience short-term psychological consequences, and among the many women who do experience longer-term psychological pain, the results can be devastating. In fact, the psychological sequelae of partner abuse can also include negative physical consequences stemming from stress and trauma (for a brief review, see Campbell, 2002). For these reasons, it is important to review some of the more recent scientific findings regarding intimate partner abuse and its consequences for women's mental health.

Walker (1984) is arguably the first investigator to observe that abused women experience a variety of psychological consequences. Since then researchers have extensively studied possible abuse correlates and have argued that partner-abused women can experience post-traumatic stress disorder (PTSD), anxiety, depression, panic, drug abuse, eating or body image disorders, and suicidal ideation (Al-Modollal, Peden, & Anderson, 2008; Campbell, 2002; Koss, Bailey, Yuan, Herrera, & Lichter, 2003; Renner & Markward, 2009). PTSD and depression appear to be the most prevalent and most researched consequences of abuse. In fact, as Warshaw et al. (2009) point out, depression and PTSD are being seen by researchers and theorists as comorbid conditions for women who experience intimate partner violence. However, there is still debate in the scientific literature as to whether PTSD and depression capture all of the mental health consequences of partner abuse (Warshaw et al., 2009).

It is also important to note that there is some evidence that abuse-precipitated mental health problems compound over the victims' lifetime and abuse episodes. The National Violence Against Women Survey (Fogarty, Fredman, Heeren, & Liebschutz, 2008) found that 36% of partner-abused women reported depression symptoms. Similarly, 35% of women who were abused as children reported depression symptoms. However, among the women who experienced abuse both as a child and later by an adult partner, 50% reported depression symptoms. This may not be such a counterintuitive finding, given that PTSD precipitates long-term, possibly permanent, changes in hormonal and physiological responses to stress and other stimuli (see Davidson & van der Kolk, 1996; Rellini, Hamilton, Delville, & Meston, 2009; Spilsbury, 2009). A woman who was abused at one time in her life may be permanently predisposed to negative psychological consequences throughout her life.

These results support the argument by Warshaw et al. (2009) that there may be something akin to a negative mental health cycle for women victims of abuse. Childhood victimization increases the odds that the woman may be victimized by an adult partner. In fact, women who are sexually or physically abused as children are six times more likely than nonabused children to experience either physical or sexual intimate partner violence in adulthood (Kimerling, Alvarez, Pavao, & Baumrind, 2007). Victimization in turn results in a greater likelihood for PTSD, depression, substance abuse, or other abuse-borne psychological consequences, which may put the victim at even greater risk for further abuse (Briere et al., 1997; Goodman et al., 1997). This vicious cycle may be compounded further by the abuser, who questions and attacks his partner's mental health within their relationship and then uses the victim's mental health in judicial proceedings against her, particularly in child custody, separation, or divorce proceedings (Warshaw, Moroney, & Barnes, 2003).

Further still, psychological violence such as treating someone as an inferior, verbal abuse, monitoring behavior (including stalking behavior), and public embarrassment also predicts long-term mental health consequences (Follingstad, 2009). For instance, being stalked by an abuser after the issuance of a protective order against him is associated with women's anxiety and psychological distress (Logan & Cole, 2007). And there is good evidence that psychological abuse acts above and beyond physical abuse, injuries, and sexual coercion in precipitating, exacerbating, and prolonging PTSD and depression (Mechanic, Weaver, & Resick, 2008). Again, there is good evidence that abuse-precipitated mental health issues can be compounding and can last much longer than a single episode.

Intimate partner sexual aggression is a stronger predictor of PTSD than physical abuse (Taft, Resick, Panuzio, Vogt, & Mechanic, 2007; Bennice, Resick, Mechanic, & Astin, 2003). Taft et al. and Bennice et al. argue that this may be the case because women who are sexually abused by their partners are more likely than physically abused women to use moving-away defense mechanisms such as avoiding friends and family, using drugs or alcohol, social withdrawal (cocooning), and self-criticism. Because moving-away defense mechanisms separate the victim from important sources of social support, the mental health consequences of intimate partner sexual abuse may tend to be longer lasting (Canady & Babcock, 2009; Taft et al, 2007). Canady and Babcock (2009) found that social withdrawal and self-criticism were especially predictive of long-term mental health issues, which further supports the theory that social withdrawal can be particularly harmful for intimate sexual abuse victims.

It is important to note that while intimate sexual aggression better predicts the long-term mental health problems than does physical assault, physical assault also predicts depression severity (Taft et al., 2007).

WHICH ABUSE VICTIMS ARE MORE LIKELY TO AVOID LONG-TERM PSYCHOLOGICAL DISTRESS?

There is good evidence (summarized by Warshaw et al., 2009) that women with better social support (e.g., supportive friends and family) are less likely to experience long-term abuse-related mental health issues. Thus, when a women is abused it is vital that the she have and use her social support. Furthermore, there are some women who definitively choose to leave or stay, as opposed to women who are in and out of a relationship with the abuser. Women who clearly and definitively decide to stay in or leave an abusive relationship tend to have better long-term psychological outcomes (Bell, Goodman, & Dutton, 2007). This may be a function of better mental health or resilience in the victim prior to the abuse. However, much of the research in this area is fairly recent, and investigators are just beginning to explore possible factors that may predict abuse victims' mental health outcomes.

TREATMENT OF ABUSE SURVIVORS

Warshaw et al. (2009) thoroughly reviewed the literature on abuse survivors' mental health and make several suggestions for clinicians and researchers. Among these suggestions are the development and trial of treatment policies that consider culture, trauma, and intimate partner violence; the inclusion of assessment for intimate partner violence during peripartum depression assessment; and development among clinical practitioners (including medical and psychological clinicians) of better understanding for the links between intimate partner violence and mental health consequences. In addition, researchers should further examine these relationships and the possible mental health consequences to better inform clinical practice.

PREVENTING ABUSE

The previous section briefly describes some of the mental health consequences for women who are abused by their partners. Although treatment for the victims is important and research in this area should continue to explore ways to better help victims, preventing abuse is also an important—and perhaps more helpful—way of avoiding the consequences of abuse and the need for treatment of its victims. Intervention with potentially abusive adolescent males may be more effective in preventing abuse than the adult postabuse interventions that are currently the norm.

Abuse is a very broad topic with a number of differing scientific, legal, and lay definitions (see Bratton, Roseman, & Schweinle, in press). Abuse can occur within families, between peers, between partners, etc. However, this chapter focuses on male-to-female intimate partner abuse in adulthood. This is because while women may abuse their male partners as often as male partners abuse their female partners (Centers for Disease Control and Prevention, 2009), women do not hit as hard as men and are not as likely to cause serious injury or other negative consequences to their partners (Balsam, Rothblum, & Beauchaine, 2005; Campbell, 2004; Dobash & Dobash, 2004; Ehrensaft, Moffitt, & Caspi, 2006; Morse, 1995; Paul, Smith, & Long, 2006; Schaefer & Caetano, 1998). Therefore, the focus of the remainder of this chapter is on prevention through intervention with at-risk adolescent boys.

It is important to focus on adolescent boys, because as they become adult men, generally from age 15 to age 25, the likelihood that they will be involved in a close relationship increases. The likelihood that a male will abuse his partner also rapidly increases during this developmental phase (O'Leary, 2000). This may be a good time to intervene in ways that may prevent partner-abusive behaviors during adulthood.

It is important to ascertain whether abusive or potentially abusive adolescent males become abusive adult males and if intervention programs actually work. If this is the case, then it is important to demonstrate whether adolescence, the time when young men are beginning to explore close relationships, might be a better developmental stage than adulthood for interventions designed to reduce adult abusiveness.

YOUNG AGGRESSORS BECOME ADULT ABUSERS

There is some scientific evidence supporting the conclusion that aggressive boys develop into abusive men. For instance, Herrenkohl, Huang, Tajima, and Whitney (2003) found that 15- to 18-year-olds who were violent toward peers were more likely to be violent toward their intimate partners in adult life. Furthermore,

Foshee, Benefield, Ennet, Bauman, and Suchindran (2004) found that physical fighting with adolescent peers predicts partner abuse during adulthood. These results suggest two things. First, adolescents who are violent toward others have a greater tendency to be violent toward their romantic partners when they become adults. Second, because of this relationship between adolescent violence and adult partner violence, it is possible to predict with some reliability which adolescent males are likely to later abuse their adult partners.

Longitudinal prospective studies further support the argument that abusive teens are more likely than nonabusive teens to become partner-abusive adults. For instance, Woodward, Fergusson, and Horwood (2002) followed a cohort of New Zealand youths from birth through age 21. The youths who behaved in an antisocial manner early in life were significantly more likely to abuse their partners later in life. Furthermore, Magdol, Moffitt, Caspi, and Silva (1998) found among a sample of 992 New Zealanders, who were tracked from birth to 21 years of age, that aggressive delinquency at age 15 was significantly predictive of partner abuse at age 21. Finally, O'Donnell, Stueve, Myint-U, Duran, Agronick, and Wilson-Simmons (2006) found similar results among an American sample when they surveyed 977 8th-graders and then resurveyed the group around their 19th birthday. Similarly, Ehrensaft et al. (2003) followed 543 children from 1975 to 1999. The children and their mothers were interviewed several times over this time span. The teens who had been abused as children, who had witnessed violence between parents, and who exhibited the most conduct-disordered behaviors while growing up were the most likely to cause injury to their partners as adults. Taken together, these results offer strong evidence that physically aggressive teens tend to become partner-abusive adults.

If we are to conclude that interventions work for teens, then we must determine whether intervention works at all. If so, then investing intervention effort on at-risk adolescents might not be the best strategy for several reasons. First, while violent adolescents are more likely to become partner-violent adults, not all will. Therefore, intervention would have to involve a larger number of adolescents in order to hopefully intervene with the ones who will become abusive adults. If, however, intervention efforts are focused specifically on the men who have demonstrated abusive behavior, then the intervention would need to be brought to a smaller number of people, which could concentrate and/or better focus the available intervention resources.

ABUSIVE MEN ARE LIKELY TO CONTINUE TO BE VIOLENT

In general, several investigators have studied the likelihood that an abusive male will stop abusing on his own or through an abuser treatment program. For instance, Feld and Straus (1990) sent questionnaires to 8,145 families over a two-year period as part of their influential and ongoing National Family Violence Survey (Straus & Gelles, 1990). This longitudinal research was designed specifically to look for changes in abusive behavior over time. Feld and Straus found that about two-thirds of men who had been physically abusive at least three times in the year before completing the first questionnaire were still abusive a year later. If we generalize these findings to the population of men at large, then the probability that an abusive man will stop abusing his wife is substantially less than a coin flip. In other words, it is reasonable to expect that a man who has been abusive will continue to be abusive. Unfortunately, Feld and Straus (1990) did not measure other forms of abuse in their sample (e.g., psychological or financial abuse). Thus, the one-third of the men in the sample who were no longer physically abusive may have stopped physical abuse and switched to or continued psychological or other forms of abuse.

O'Leary et al. (1989) conducted a similar longitudinal study of 272 newly married couples. Similar to the Feld and Straus (1990) findings, almost two-thirds (65%) of the men in the sample who were physically violent before the marriage also physically abused their wives in the two and a half years following the first interview. Again, no data were collected about the men's psychological and other nonphysical forms of abuse. However, the results were clear: only about 1 in 3 physically abusive men stop physically abusing their wives.

In a similar longitudinal design, Quigley and Leonard (1996) followed 188 newly married couples in which the husband had been physically abusive of his fiancée in the previous year. The engaged partners completed their questionnaires separately and submitted them separately by mail. The couples were also paid separately for completing and returning the questionnaires. This process was repeated one year into the couples' marriages and again at three years into their marriages. While the most violent men were the least likely to stop being violent, the minimally violent men in this sample still had a two out of three chance of continuing their violence in the second and third years of the marriage. While it is possible that an abusive husband will stop being violent, the chance that he will is very low.

The studies mentioned above did not investigate forms of abuse other than physical. Aldarondo (1996), however, in his three-year study of 772 married couples extended previous work by looking into the husbands' emotional abuse of their wives. Interestingly, all of the husbands who were physically violent in the first year of the study continued to be emotionally abusive in the second and third years. So, even if the man stopped physically assaulting his wife, he continued to abuse her emotionally during the second and third years of their marriage. This finding answers questions left by other studies in that it suggests that abusive men who stop physically abusing their wives are likely to keep abusing them emotionally.

Jacobson and Gottman (1998) further extended this line of research by looking into men's systematic use of intimidation (e.g., physical, emotional, etc.) to control their female partners. This study involved a sample of 140 married couples over two years. This is a much deeper look at couples with an abusive husband because it included the spouses' physiological (i.e., polygraph-type) reactions as well as videotape analysis of the spouses' facial expressions and other interaction behaviors while the husband and wife discussed a problematic marital issue. In summary, while 54% of the men in the sample reduced their physical violence during the two-year course of the study, only 7% of the men completely stopped being physically violent over the two-year time frame. Jacobson and Gottman argue that the reduction in physical violence by some of the men may have been replaced by emotional abuse, because once the man had established dominance and control, he could use less extreme abuse methods (e.g., emotional or financial abuse) that were not likely to result in incarceration.

Interestingly, Jacobson and Gottman (1998) found that among the men who stopped being violent or became less physically violent, nothing that the women did appeared to explain why the men stopped their abusive behavior. It therefore stands to reason that only characteristics of the abusers themselves predict whether the violence will decrease or ultimately stop.

So, are violent men likely to continue to be violent? The answer is yes; an abusive adult male will probably continue to be abusive over the course of and across his relationship(s). Findings across several studies support the old adage among psychologists that the best predictor of future behavior is past behavior. It also appears that if an abusive adult male reduces or ceases his physical violence, then the often-accompanying emotional abuse will continue or will take the place of physical assault in the man's pursuit of control and domination in his marriage.

ADULT ABUSER TREATMENT PROGRAMS

Several batterer programs have been created and are used in state and military criminal justice settings. The following discussion is based on the work of Babcock, Green, and Robie (2004); Gondolf (2002, 2009); and Roberts (2002). Both Gondolf and Roberts described several of the various batterer treatment programs that have been developed. Babcock et al. conducted a meta-analysis of the effectiveness of these programs in halting men's abusive behavior. It is important to point out that batterer intervention programs (BIPs), whether voluntary or court mandated, are essentially after-the-fact attempts to reduce wife abuse. In other words, these programs are for men who have already demonstrated their abusive nature.

The Duluth Model (Paymar, 1993; Pence & Paymar, 1993) is perhaps the most widely used BIP in the United States. The Duluth Model is built on the idea that abusive men abuse their partners to achieve and maintain power and control in the relationship. Perhaps you have seen the Power and Control Wheel developed by Pence and Paymar (1993). This wheel diagrams the central theory of the Duluth Model, which focuses on stopping the abuse immediately and on changing men's attitudes that abusive behavior is okay. (Note that there is a positive relationship between attitudes that are permissive of abuse and actual abuse; see Schwartz, O'Leary, & Kendziora, 1997). Duluth Model practitioners combine parts of several different approaches to try to change abusive men's attitudes toward women and abusive behavior.

Another BIP approach is based in psychodynamic theory (Browne & Saunders, 1997; Dutton, 1998; Stosny, 1995). Psychodynamic treatment focuses on the personality of the abuser and holds that men's abusive behavior is the product of the men's life experiences from birth to the present. Psychodynamic abuser therapy includes offering abusive men positive support and the camaraderie of other men through group sessions. Because there is an important association between insecure attachment and abuse (for an interview, see Dutton, 1998), these sessions are designed to help the abuser become better able to attach or emotionally bond to his partner and, as a result, have less fearful nonabusive relationships.

There are other approaches, including anger management and couples counseling (Geffner & Mantooth, 2000). One problem with anger management is the possible inference that the abuser is somehow provoked by the victim. This is simply not the case (see Schweinle & Ickes, 2007; Schweinle, Ickes, & Bernstein, 2002; Schweinle, Ickes, Rollings, & Jacquot, 2010). By treating partner abuse as a relationship problem, couples therapy also implies that the victim is perhaps partially to blame for the abusive behavior and that both partners— the abuser and the victim—need to work together to stop the abuse. Again, this is a false assumption because recent findings have demonstrated that abusiveness is a characteristic of the abuser, not of the victim. Worse still, couples therapy places the woman in close contact with her abuser to discuss potentially explosive relationship issues. This is inherently risky.

Babcock et al. (2004) conducted a thorough meta-analysis of 22 scientific articles on the effectiveness of batterer treatment program effectiveness. The treatment programs reviewed included the Duluth Model, cognitive behavior therapy, anger management, probation, and other abuser treatment modalities. The experimental methods included quasi- and true-experimental designs. Unfortunately, Babcock et al. found that the recidivism rates for the abusers who were treated were very similar to the recidivism rates for men who were not treated at all. Furthermore, the differences between treatment types (e.g., Duluth Model vs. cognitive behavior therapy) were not significant. Finally, Babcock et al. summarize that the likelihood that a treated batterer will reabuse is about 40%, whereas for a nontreated batterer it is about 35%. In summary, Babcock et al. found that abuser treatment programs are not very effective in stopping abuse.

Jackson et al. (2003) conducted a similar but smaller review of two BIP effectiveness research programs for the National Institute of Justice. These studies compared Duluth Model treatment and cognitive behavioral therapy to probation alone. One program was in Broward County, Florida; the other was in Brooklyn, New York. The findings were startling. Generally speaking, neither of the BIPs was much more effective than probation alone. In fact, in Broward County the men who were assigned to the BIP were slightly more likely to abuse their partners again than the men who were only given probation.

BIPs are built on reasonable psychological theory and follow rational assumptions that seem to explain why men abuse and what can be done to stop the abuse. Unfortunately, however, the only reasonable conclusion that can be drawn from the research reviewed here is that we are unlikely to stop an adult abuser from abusing. Of course, there are anecdotal cases of abusive men who have stopped either in treatment or on their own. And these cases may, by themselves, justify the use of batterer treatment. Statistically speaking, however, these are exceptional cases. The vast majority of abusive men do not stop abusing within and across their close relationships, and BIPs are generally not very effective. Given these sobering conclusions, it seems reasonable to direct attention to other possible ways of preventing partner abuse, such as intervention during adolescence.

INTERVENTION IN ADOLESCENCE FOR ABUSIVE TEENS

Peer dating violence has significant negative consequences on the mental health of victims. For instance, Banyard and Cross (2008) recently found that victims of dating violence tended to experience more depression and diminished academic performance. (This relationship appears to be further complicated by substance abuse, though the causal pathways are as yet unclear.) Regardless, for these reasons alone it is important to prevent or stop partner violence between teens. However, intervention with abusive adolescents may have the long-term effect of helping prevent abusive behavior in adulthood.

It stands to reason that if most abusive adult men will not or cannot be made to stop abusing, there might be an earlier developmental period during potentially (or actively) abusive men's lives when the abuse could be prevented or stopped. Several investigators have made this argument based on sound theory and research (Avery-Leaf, Cascardi, O'Leary, & Cano, 1997; Banyard & Cross, 2008; Ehrensaft et al., 2003; Magdol et al., 1998). The following paragraphs describe these arguments as they developed (i.e., in chronological order) and indicate that intervention with abusive and potentially abusive male teens may be a more effective short- and long-term approach to preventing (at least) some abusive behavior during and after adolescence.

Avery-Leaf et al. (1997) reported on a five-session dating violence training program that they developed and tested among 192 New York high school students. The program, which focused on changing the students' attitudes toward acceptance of partner violence, resulted in a significant reduction in the male students' acceptance of and justification for dating violence. However, on the one hand there is a psychologically murky and unreliable relationship between peoples' attitudes and their actual behavior (for a recent and well-written overview of this topic, see Albarracin, Johnson, & Zanna, 2009). So, it would be a shaky leap of logic to conclude that the five-session program resulted in less actual partner violence.

On the other hand, Schwartz et al. (1997) found a significant relationship specifically between young males' attitudes toward aggression (i.e., their justification of aggression) and actual aggression. This does support the conclusion that the program developed by Avery-Leaf et al. (1997) does effectively reduce teen dating violence. By extension, and based on the relationship between teen and adult partner violence described above, it is reasonable to conclude that this brief five-session intervention will result in at least some reduction in adult partner violence for the students who participated.

As part of the longitudinal study discussed earlier in this chapter, Magdol et al. (1998) looked into the possible early childhood, late childhood, and adolescent markers for partner abuse in adulthood. Among the significant predictors, a close relationship between the adolescent and his parent was negatively associated with adult partner abuse. Furthermore, having parents with higher-status occupations while a boy is in middle school and having both parents living in the household were negatively associated with adult partner abuse. Positive childhood predictors of adult partner abuse included dropping out of school and delinquency in adolescence.

Considering that it is possible to identify potential adult abusers during their middle school years, it may be reasonable to argue that identifying at-risk middle school males and intervening with them while they are in middle school would be a good approach. However, the reliability of the middle school–age predictors is somewhat less than that of high school–age predictors. In other words, it is more difficult to predict a person's behavior the longer the time between the prediction and when you anticipate the behavior occurring. Therefore, identifying at-risk boys during middle school and intervening may not be cost-effective, because intervention would have to involve a very large group of boys in order to have the expectation of bringing about results. Based on this, Magdol et al. (1998) argue that early adolescence (i.e., early high school age), would be a better time to intervene, because as time lengthens between an intervention and the focal outcome behavior, the efficacy of the intervention wanes (Caspi & Bem, 1990). In other words, intervention when the early adolescent males are closer to exploring and entering close relationships would be more effective in preventing teen partner abuse and, theoretically, adult partner abuse.

Ehrensaft et al. (2003) argued on the basis of their findings from the Children in Communities Study that partner violence prevention strategies should focus on children with a history of abuse by parents and other adults and that these strategies should focus on avoiding escalation of behavioral problems. Ehrensaft et al. cite social learning theory and research to conclude that children who witness abuse between parents can be helped to understand that violence is not an acceptable or effective means of handling conflict in close relationships. In other words, children who grow up learning that violence is a normal or acceptable means of conflict resolution can learn nonviolent conflict resolution methods. Ehrensaft et al. further suggest that these prevention programs could be coordinated with courts, law enforcement, and services for abused women and children.

However, in contrast to Avery-Leaf et al. (1997) and Magdol et al. (1998), Ehrensaft et al. (2003) argue that prevention should occur earlier than adolescence (i.e., in late childhood) so that abusive responses to conflict do not become entrenched in the child's psyche and behavior patterns and then later emerge in adolescent and adult close relationships. Ehrensaft et al. base this argument on their clinical observation that excessive punishment by parents is difficult to extinguish by the time a child becomes an adolescent. Therefore, intervention should occur while the child is younger and has not necessarily been taught to resolve relationship conflict through extreme coercive methods.

In summary, there are both theoretical arguments and a few empirical findings that support the conclusion that partner-abuse intervention with adolescent boys should occur sometime earlier than in adulthood. However, the optimal time for such intervention is under debate in the research literature. Some researchers argue that early middle school (i.e., preadolescence) would be optimal. Other investigators argue that intervention in early adolescence, when the boys are first exploring close relationships, would be better. Further research is needed in this area to assess the effectiveness of adolescent abuse intervention and to better pinpoint the optimal developmental stage for such intervention.

CONCLUSION

There is some direct evidence that an abusive teen will mature into an abusive adult. The research to date tends to suggest that an abusive adult man will continue to be abusive to his partner whether or not he ever participates in a BIP. However, there is some preliminary evidence that intervention with abusive and potentially abusive boys will reduce the likelihood that they will be abusive toward their partners in adulthood. Taken together, these results suggest that partner-abuse prevention might be more effectively focused on adolescent males before they become adult abusers who are highly resistant to nonpunitive intervention. Future research should focus on the development of early interventions for young men. More distal research should longitudinally explore the short- and long-term effectiveness of such intervention programs.

REFERENCES

Albarracin, D. Johnson, B., & Zanna, M. (2009). *The handbook of attitudes.* Mahwah, NJ: Erlbaum.

Aldarondo, E. (1996). Cessation and persistence of wife assault. *American Journal of Orthopsychiatry, 66,* 141–151.

Al-Modallal, H., Peden, A., & Anderson, D. (2008). Impact of physical abuse on adulthood depressive symptoms among women. *Issues in Mental Health Nursing, 29,* 299–314.

Archer, J. (2000). Sex differences in aggression between heterosexual partners: A meta-analytic review. *Psychological Bulletin, 26,* 651–680.

Avery-Leaf, S., Cascardi, M., O'Leary, K., & Cano, A. (1997). Efficacy of dating violence prevention program on attitudes justifying aggression. *Journal of Adolescent Health, 21,* 11–17.

Babcock, J., Green, C., & Robie, C. (2004). Does batterer treatment work? A meta-analytic review of domestic violence treatment. *Clinical Psychology Review, 23,* 1023–1053.

Balsam, K., Rothblum, E., & Beauchaine, T. (2005). Victimization over lifespan: A comparison of lesbian, gay, and heterosexual siblings. *Journal of Consulting and Clinical Psychology, 73,* 477–487.

Banyard, V., & Cross, C. (2008). Consequences of teen dating violence. *Violence Against Women, 14,* 998–1013.

Bell, M., Goodman, L., & Dutton, M. (2007). The dynamics of staying and leaving: Implications for battered women's emotional well being and experiences of violence at the end of the year. *Journal of Family Violence, 22,* 413–428.

Bennice, J., Resick, P., Mechanic, M., & Astin, M. (2003). The relative effects of intimate partner physical and sexual violence on post-traumatic stress disorder symptomatology. *Violence and Victims, 18,* 87–94.

Bratton, I., Roseman, C., & Schweinle, W. (in press). Educating teens to discriminate abusive from non-abusive situations. In M. Paludi (Ed.), *The psychology of teen violence and victimization.* Santa Barbara, CA: Praeger.

Briere, J., Woo, R., McRae, B., Foltz, J., & Sitzman, R. (1997). Lifetime victimization history, demographics, and clinical status in female psychiatric emergency room patients. *Journal of Nervous and Mental Disease, 185,* 95–101.

Browne, K., & Saunders, D. (1997). Process-psychodynamic groups for men who batter: A brief treatment model. *Families in Society, 78,* 265–272.

Campbell, J. (2002). Health consequences of intimate partner violence. *Lancet, 359,* 1331–1336.

Campbell, J. (2004). Helping women understand their risk in situations of partner violence. *Journal of Interpersonal Violence, 19,* 1464–167.

Canady, B., & Babcock, J. (2009). The protective functions of social support and coping for women experiencing intimate partner abuse. *Journal of Aggression, Maltreatment and Trauma, 18,* 443–458.

Caspi, A., & Bem, D. (1990). Personality continuity and change across the life course. In L. Pervin (Ed.), *Handbook of personality: Theory and research* (pp. 549–575). New York: Guilford.

Centers for Disease Control and Prevention (2003). *Costs of intimate partner violence against women in the United States.* Atlanta, GA: Author.

Centers for Disease Control and Prevention (2009). Youth Risk Behavioral Surveillance System (2009). Retrieved on October 13, 2010, from http://www.cdc.gov/mmwr/pdf/ss/ss5905.pdf.

Davidson, J., & van der Kolk, B. (1996). The psychopharmacological treatment of post-traumatic stress disorder. In B. van der Kolk & L. Weisaeth (Eds.), *Traumatic stress: The effects of overwhelming experience on mind, body, and society* (pp. 510–524). New York: Guilford.

Dobash, R. P., & Dobash, R. E. (2004). Women's violence to men in intimate relationships—Working on a puzzle. *British Journal of Criminology, 44,* 324–349.

Dutton, D. (1998). *The abusive personality: Violence and control in intimate relationships.* New York: Guilford.

Ehrensaft, M., Cohen, P., Brown, J., Smailes, E., Chen, H., & Johnson, J. (2003). Intergenerational transmission of partner violence: A 20-year prospective study. *Journal of Consulting and Clinical Psychology, 71,* 741–753.

Ehrensaft, M., Moffitt, T., & Caspi, A. (2006). Is domestic violence followed by an increased risk of psychiatric disorders among women but not men? A longitudinal cohort study. *American Journal of Psychiatry, 163,* 885–892.

Feld, S., & Straus, M. (1990). Escalation and desistence from wife assault. In M. Straus & R. Gelles (Eds.), *Physical violence in American families: Risk factors and adaptations to violence in 8,145 families* (pp. 489–505). New Brunswick, NJ: Transaction Publishers.

Fogarty, C., Fredman, I., Heeren, T., & Liebschutz, J. (2008). Synergystic effects of child abuse and intimate partner violence on depressive symptoms in women. *Preventive Medicine, 46,* 463–469.

Follingstad, D. (2009). The impact of psychological aggression on women's mental health and behavior. *Trauma, Violence, and Abuse, 10,* 271–289.

Foshee, V., Benefield, T., Ennett, S., Bauman, K., & Suchindran, C. (2004). Longitudinal predictors of serious physical and sexual dating violence victimization during adolescence. *Preventive Medicine, 39,* 1007–1016.

Geffner, R., & Mantooth, C. (2000). *Ending spouse/partner abuse: A psychoeducational approach for individuals and couples.* New York: Springer.

Gondolf, E. (2002). *Batterer intervention systems.* Thousand Oaks, CA: Sage.

Gondolf, E. (2009). Outcomes from referring batterer program participants to mental health treatment. *Journal of Family Violence, 24,* 577–588.

Goodman L., Dutton M., & Harris M. (1997). The relationship between violence dimensions and symptom severity among homeless, mentally ill women. *Journal of Traumatic Stress, 10,* 51–70.

Herrenkohl, T., Huang, B., Tajima, E., & Whitney, S. (2003). Examining the link between child abuse and youth violence. *Journal of Interpersonal Violence, 18,* 1189–1208.

Jackson, S., Feder, L., Forde, D. R., Davis, R. C. Maxwell, C. D., & Taylor, B. G. (2003). *Batterer intervention programs: Where do we go from here?* NCJ Publication No. NCJ 195079. Washington, DC: U.S. Government Printing Office.

Jacobson, N., & Gottman, J. (1998). *When men batter women: New insights into ending abusive relationships.* New York: Simon & Schuster.

Kimerling, R., Alvarez, J., Pavao, J. & Baumrind, N. (2007). Epidemiology and consequences of women's revictimization. *Women's Health Issues, 17,* 101–106.

Koss, M., Bailey, J., Yuan, N., Herrera, V., & Lichter, E. (2003). Depression and PTSD in survivors of male violence: Research and training initiatives to facilitate recovery. *Psychology of Women Quarterly, 27,* 130–142.

Koss, M., Goodman, L., & Browne, L. (1994). *No safe haven: Male violence against women at home, at work, and in the community.* Washington, DC: American Psychological Association.

Logan, T. K., & Cole, J. (2007). The impact of partner stalking on mental health and protective order outcomes over time. *Violence and Victims, 22,* 546–562.

Magdol, L., Moffitt, T., Caspi, A., & Silva, P. (1998). Developmental antecedents of partner abuse: A prospective longitudinal study. *Journal of Abnormal Psychology, 107,* 375–389.

Mechanic, M., Weaver, T., & Resick, P. (2008). Mental health consequences of intimate partner abuse: A multidimensional assessment of four different forms of abuse. *Violence Against Women, 14,* 634–654.

Morse, B. (1995). Beyond the Conflict Tactics Scale: Assessing gender differences in partner violence. *Violence and Victims, 10,* 251–272.

O'Donnell, L., Stueve, A., Myint-U, A., Duran, R., Agronick, G., & Wilson-Simmons, R. (2006). Middle school aggression and subsequent intimate partner physical violence. *Journal of Youth and Adolescence, 35,* 693–703.

O'Leary, D., Barling, J., Arias, I., Rosenbaum, A., Malone, J., & Tyree, A. (1989). Prevalence and stability of physical aggression between spouses: A longitudinal analysis. *Journal of Consulting and Clinical Psychology, 57,* 263–268.

O'Leary, K. (2000). Are women really more aggressive than men in intimate relationships? [Comment on Archer (2000).] *Psychological Bulletin, 126,* 685–689.

Paul, G., Smith, S., & Long, J. (2006). Experience of intimate partner violence among women and men attending general practices in Dublin, Ireland: A cross-sectional survey. *European Journal of General Practice, 12,* 66–69.

Paymar, M. (1993). *Violent no more: Helping men end domestic abuse.* Alameda, CA: Hunter House.

Pence, E., & Paymar, M. (1993). *Education groups for men who batter: The Duluth Model.* New York: Springer.

Quigley, B., & Leonard, K. (1996). Desistance from marital violence in the early years of marriage. *Violence and Victims, 11,* 355–370.

Rellini, A., Hamilton, L., Delville, Y., & Meston, C. (2009) The cortisol response during physiological sexual arousal in adult women with a history of childhood sexual abuse. *Journal of Traumatic Stress, 22,* 557–565.

Renner, L., & Markward, M. (2009). Factors associated with suicidal ideation among women abused in intimate partner relationships. *Smith College Studies in Social Work, 79,* 139–154.

Roberts, A. (Ed.). (2002). *Handbook of domestic violence intervention strategies.* New York: Oxford University Press.

Schaefer, J., & Caetano, R. (1998). Rates of intimate partner violence in the United States. *American Journal of Public Health, 110,* 1702–1705.

Schwartz, M., O'Leary, S., & Kendziora, K. (1997). Dating aggression among high school students. *Violence and Victims, 12,* 295–305.

Schweinle, W., & Ickes, W. (2007). The role of men's critical/rejecting overattribution bias, affect and attentional disengagement in marital aggression. *Journal of Social and Clinical Psychology, 26,* 175–199.

Schweinle, W., Ickes, W., & Bernstein, I. (2002). Empathic inaccuracy in husband to wife aggression: The overattribution bias. *Personal Relationships, 9,* 141–158.

Schweinle, W., Ickes, W., Rollings, K., and Jacquot, C. (2010). Maritally aggressive men: Angry, egocentric, impulsive and/or biased. *Journal of Language and Social Psychology, 29,* 399–424.

Spilsbury, J. C. (2009). Sleep as a mediator in the pathway from violence-induced traumatic stress to poorer health and functioning: A review of the literature and proposed conceptual model. *Behavioral Sleep Medicine, 7,* 223–244.

Stosny, S. (1995). *Treating attachment abuse: A compassion approach.* New York: Springer.

Straus, M., & Gelles, R. (1990). *Physical violence in American families: Risk factors and adaptations to violence in 8,145 families.* New Brunswick, NJ: Transaction Publishers.

Taft, C., Resick, P., Panuzio, J., Vogt, D., & Mechanic, M. (2007). Coping among victims of relationship abuse: A longitudinal examination. *Violence and Victims, 22,* 408–418.

Walker, L. (1984). *The battered woman syndrome.* New York: Springer.

Warshaw, C., Brashler, P., & Gil, J. (2009). Mental health consequences of intimate partner violence. In C. Mitchell & D. Anglin (Eds.), *Intimate partner violence: A health-based perspective* (pp. 147–171). New York: Oxford University Press.

Warshaw, C., Moroney, G., & Barnes, H. (2003). *Report on mental health issues and service needs in Chicago-area domestic violence programs.* Chicago: Domestic Violence and Mental Health Policy Initiative.

Woodward, L., Fergusson, D., & Horwood, L. (2002). Romantic relationships of young people with childhood and adolescent onset antisocial behavior problems. *Journal of Abnormal Child Psychology, 30,* 231–243.

Chapter 9

Intimate Partner Violence during Adolescence

Emilio Ulloa, Vanessa Watts, Monica Ulibarri, Donna Castañeda, and Audrey Hokoda

DEFINITIONS OF INTIMATE PARTNER VIOLENCE AMONG ADOLESCENT GIRLS

Intimate partner violence among adolescents has been defined as "any attempt to control or dominate another person physically, sexually, or psychologically, causing some level of harm" (Wekerle and Wolfe, 1999, p. 436). More specifically, according to the Centers for Disease Control and Prevention (2009), physical abuse refers to instances in which a partner is hit, pinched, shoved, or kicked with the intention to harm, disable, or even kill. Sexual abuse refers to instances in which a partner is forced to engage in a sex act when she does not or cannot give consent, whether or not the act is completed, and also refers to noncontact sexual abuse, such as verbal sexual harassment. Psychological abuse, which includes emotional abuse, refers to threatening a partner or harming her sense of self-worth and can include shaming, bullying, or embarrassing a partner on purpose; name calling; and keeping the partner away from friends and family. These categories of aggression in relationships can be described separately, which is useful, but they are related to each other and often co-occur in specific relationships among adolescents (Cano, Avery-Leaf, Cascardi, & O'Leary, 1998; O'Leary & Smith Slep, 2003;

Ozer Tschann, Pasch, & Flores, 2004; Silverman, Raj, Mucci, & Hathaway, 2001). Likewise, among adolescents, being a perpetrator of intimate partner violence is associated with being a victim of intimate partner violence (Bennett & Fineran, 1998; Gaertner & Foshee, 1999; Gray & Foshee, 1997; Malik, Sorenson, & Aneshensel, 1997; O'Leary, Smith Slep, Avery-Leaf, & Cascardi, 2008; Simon, Miller, Gorman-Smith, Orpinas, & Sullivan, 2010). Finally, research indicates high stability across time in dating violence perpetration and victimization among both girls and boys in high school dating couples (O'Leary & Smith Slep, 2003).

Understanding intimate partner violence among adolescents has expanded to include stalking behavior in the context of dating relationships (Coker, Sanderson, Cantu, Huerta, & Fadden, 2008) and romantic relational aggression, or behaviors that harm by damaging the romantic relationship (Linder, Crick, & Collins, 2002) such as flirting with another to anger the partner or threatening to leave the relationship if a partner does not comply. Furthermore, the unprecedented expansion of cell phone technology, social networking sites, email, and Internet chat has opened up new avenues for social interactions and relationships and consequently for intimate partner violence among adolescents. Types of abuse that employ these technologies include sending threatening and/or insulting messages via email or text messaging; excessive text messaging or phone calls in an attempt to keep tabs on a partner; checking a partner's phone logs, texts, email, and web browsing histories; and posting insults or defamatory information on a partner's Facebook or Myspace profile page. Nonetheless, while these technological advances provide new possibilities through which dating violence can occur, such technologically mediated behavior may not necessarily be defined by adolescents themselves as forms of dating violence and may hold to a traditional definition of dating violence as physical violence that happens in face-to-face situations (Baker & Helm, 2010).

Another definitional issue among adolescents is that the terminology applied to describe physical, sexual, and psychological abuse varies quite a bit. For example, the Centers for Disease Control and Prevention uses the term "intimate partner violence" to describe violence across adults and adolescents but also makes use of the term "teen dating violence" when referring specifically to adolescents (Centers for Disease Control and Prevention, 2009). Other terminology sometimes used to refer to violence in adolescent relationships include teen relationship violence, aggression, or abuse; courtship violence; and dating abuse, violence, or aggression (Centers for Disease Control and Prevention, n.d.; Teten, Ball, Valle, Noonan, & Rosenbluth, 2009). The variety in terminology is a concern because inconsistent terminology may serve to highlight some aspects of violence in the relationships of adolescent girls while hiding others by referring to physical, sexual, or psychological abuse either singly or in any combination (Centers for Disease Control and Prevention, n.d.; Teten et al., 2009). These terms also imply that violence occurs within the context of an ongoing close relationship. Such an assumption may be accurate for adults but can obscure the causes, patterns, and dynamics of relationship violence among adolescents. Adolescent relationships do not necessarily mirror those of adults; for instance, adolescent relationships may be long term or quite short in duration, and the partner may or may not be considered close. The partners may or may not engage in traditional dating behavior. Adolescents, particularly those who are younger and do not drive, for example, may only see their partners in school or at a park after school (see Hickman, Jaycox, & Aronoff, 2004).

PERPETRATORS/VICTIMS OF DATING VIOLENCE

Another characteristic of adolescent dating violence that may differ from domestic violence in adults is that there is a high prevalence of relationships whereby adolescents report being both victims and perpetrators of dating violence. In fact, most of the work on teen violence prevention and intervention is conceptualized for the one-sided violent relationship and thus is not focused on mutually combative relationships. Although there is sufficient research to suggest that a partner's aggression is an important predictor of one's own dating aggression, the study of co-occurring perpetration and victimization has not received as much attention. Research on dating violence in adolescence has been heavily influenced by the adult domestic violence literature and understandably focuses on men's use of violence, power, and control toward women. This is noteworthy not only because it ignores female-to-male aggression but also because research findings indicate that most adolescent violent relationships are reported to be mutually violent (e.g., Gray & Foshee, 1997; Henton, Cate, Koval, Lloyd, & Christopher, 1983; Pederson & Thomas, 1992). The phenomenon has been described as mutually combative relationships, mutually violent relationships, and dyadic patterns of aggression or has been studied as the correlation between victimization and perpetration. Gray and Foshee (1997), for example, reported on the differences between what they describe as one-sided versus mutually violent profiles. Their conclusions are disturbing. Most teens who report violence (66%) are involved in mutually violent relationships. Furthermore, teens in mutually violent relationships are more likely to experience and perpetrate more severe forms of violence and abuse and to incur injuries compared to those who report being victims or perpetrators only. In a study by Billingham (1987), 535 college students participated in a survey study that yielded similar findings. After comparing subscale scores from the Conflict Tactics Scale (Straus, 1979), Billingham discovered that participants who were categorized as being involved in mutually violent relationships used more severe forms of physical violence in their relationships compared to other groups. Renner and Whitney's (2010) study of young adult dating violence echoed these results. They found that 54% of their violent sample reported bidirectional violence, compared to the 21% and 24% who reported perpetration or victimization only, respectively.

Additionally, little is understood about patterns of violence. Girls who are involved in a mutually violent relationship are more likely to have been victims across different relationships (Gray & Foshee, 1997). This finding suggests that for some teens, dating violence is not a one-time event but instead may represent a pattern of relationships that are at high risk for violence. Mutually violent relationships may also be a reflection of the context in which aggression occurs. O'Leary and Smith Slep (2003) stress the importance of taking into account the dyadic contextual factors that lead to aggression in relationships. They call attention to the fact that relationship violence most often occurs in the context of an argument between couples (e.g., Cascardi & Vivian, 1995). O'Leary and Smith Slep (2003) posit that this line of research suggests that relative to domestic violence research, research with adolescents needs to be more focused on the effect that a partner's aggression has on the perpetration of a teen's own aggression. More research is needed to investigate teen dyadic and contextual factors in mutually violent relationships.

Despite problems associated with varying terminology used to describe violence in adolescent relationships, in this chapter we use the terms "intimate partner violence" and "dating violence" interchangeably. These are currently the terms most frequently used to describe violence in adolescent relationships and are the most descriptive of the phenomena that we discuss. As Teten et al. (2009) recommend, we refer to specific types of violence when the research indicates such behavior.

PREVALENCE OF INTIMATE PARTNER VIOLENCE AMONG ADOLESCENT GIRLS

Research on the prevalence of intimate partner violence among adolescent girls reveals that intimate partner violence is common, but rates vary widely across studies. For instance, in their comprehensive review of dating violence, Hickman et al. (2004) found that among single studies, estimates of physical victimization among girls ranged from 8% to 57%, compared to 6% to 38% among boys, while for sexual victimization estimates ranged from 14% to 43% for girls, compared to .3% to 36% for boys. Estimates of physical perpetration for girls ranged from 28% to 33%, compared to 11% to 20% for boys, while for sexual perpetration estimates for girls ranged from 2% to 24%, compared to 3% to 37% for boys. More recent research using both probability and nonprobability samples provides continuing evidence that intimate partner violence among adolescent girls, both as victims and as perpetrators, is unsettlingly common both in the United States and internationally (e.g., Antônio & Hokoda, 2009; Hokoda, Galvan, Malcarne, Castañeda, & Ulloa, 2007; Kelly, Cheng, Peralez-Dieckmann, & Martinez, 2009; Marquart, Nannini, Edwards, Stanley, & Wayman, 2007; Muñoz-Rivas, Graña, O'Leary, & González, 2007; O'Leary et al., 2008; Raiford, Wingood, & DiClemente, 2008; Rivera-Rivera, Allen-Leigh, Rodríguez-Ortega, Chavez-Ayala, & Lazcano-Ponce, 2007; Whitaker, Haileyesus, Swahn, & Saltzman, 2007; Wolitzky-Taylor et al., 2008). Even at younger ages (e.g., girls in the sixth grade who report having a boyfriend), the prevalence of intimate partner violence is high, with girls reporting a dating violence victimization rate of 27.4%, compared to 53.7% among males, and a dating violence perpetration rate of 31.5%, compared to 26.4% among boys (Simon et al., 2010).

National-level probability studies tend to provide lower estimates of intimate partner violence among adolescents. For example, the National Crime Victimization Survey (NCVS) conducted by the Department of Justice indicates that during 2001–2005, the average annual nonfatal victimization rate from intimate partners for girls aged 12–15 was 1.6%, while for boys in the same age group it was .2%. The rate increased for older adolescents aged 16–19, but girls continue to report a higher rate of victimization by an intimate partner (6.3%) than boys (0.6%) (Catalano, 2007). Another national data source, the Youth Risk Behavior Surveillance System (YRBSS), is a school-based survey conducted by the Centers for Disease Control and Prevention every two years among high school students in grades 9 to 12. The YRBSS covers six categories of health risk behavior, including violence, with one question on dating violence and another on forced sexual intercourse. The question on dating violence asks if an individual has been "hit, slapped, or physically hurt on purpose by their boyfriend or girlfriend during the 12 months before the survey." Unlike the NCVS, from 1999 to 2009 rates for victimization by a girlfriend or boyfriend among high school girls and boys in the YRBSS were quite similar and ranged from 8.8% to 9.8% for girls and 8.3% to 11% for boys. Although the rate decreased for boys in 2009 to 10.3%, the rate for girls remained stable at 9.3% (Centers for Disease Control and Prevention, 2008; National Youth Risk Behavior Study, 2009). On the other hand, girls (10.5%) were twice as likely as boys (4.5%) to report that they had ever been physically forced to have sexual intercourse (National Youth Risk Behavior Study, 2009). Likewise, with regard to the most extreme consequence of intimate partner violence, data from the Department of Justice, Bureau of Justice Statistics (Fox & Zawitz, n.d.), indicate that 5% of homicides of girls aged 12–17 are perpetrated by an intimate partner, while less than .5% of boys in that age group are killed by an intimate partner. Girls are also more likely than boys to experience physical injuries (cuts, bruises, black eyes, etc.) and to need medical attention or hospitalization from dating violence (Foshee, 1996; Muñoz-Rivas et al., 2007), although some research with adolescents shows no difference in the need for medical attention due to injury from a dating partner (O'Leary et al., 2008).

Across studies, emotional (or verbal) abuse tends to show the highest rates both for perpetration and victimization among adolescent girls, followed by physical abuse, where rates for perpetration and victimization tend to show the most variability across studies, with sexual abuse generally showing the lowest rates, particularly for sexual violence perpetration by adolescent girls (Freedner, Freed, Yang, & Austin, 2002; Hokoda et al., 2007; Ozer et al., 2004; Seligowski & West, 2009; Silverman et al., 2001). Likewise, across the three types of intimate partner violence, less severe violence shows higher prevalence rates compared to severe types of violence, particularly violence in which an object or weapon is used against a partner (Wolitzky-Taylor et al., 2008). In fact, girls tend to be less likely than boys to use an object or weapon against a partner (Simon et al., 2010).

The wide range in prevalence estimates across studies of intimate partner violence listed above (e.g., .2% to 57%) can be attributed to a number of methodological issues, such as differing types of abuse that are assessed, use of different measurement tools, conflation of social class with ethnicity/race in study design, use of population versus convenience samples, lifetime versus time-limited prevalence, sample self-selection bias and social desirability demands, one-sided versus mutual violence profiles, and even the effect of regional variations (Dutton & Hemphill, 1992; Foshee & Matthew, 2007; Gray & Foshee, 1997; Lewis & Fremouw, 2001; Marquart et al., 2007). These methodological issues notwithstanding, intimate partner violence, in the form of physical, sexual, and psychological violence, is clearly prevalent among adolescent girls in the United States.

A final issue with respect to prevalence of intimate partner violence among adolescent girls is the common finding of similarity in rates of perpetration and victimization of dating violence across girls and boys. As mentioned above, this similarity is more often found in studies of adolescent intimate partner violence compared to those among adults, where women tend to have a higher prevalence of victimization and men a higher prevalence of perpetration. In fact, in many studies adolescent girls show higher rates of dating violence perpetration than adolescent boys (e.g., Foshee, 1996; Malik et al., 1997; Muñoz-Rivas et al., 2007; O'Leary et al., 2008). Recent thinking about this phenomenon suggests that caveats other than the methodological issues mentioned above must be taken into consideration. First, the general assumption that girl violence is increasing and that girls are becoming more like boys in their use of violence may be inaccurate (Mikel Brown, Chesney-Lind, & Stein, 2007). Mikel Brown et al. make the case that girls' violence has not increased; in fact, national data systems demonstrate that arrests for girls for violent crimes have actually decreased, and their rate of violence victimization has decreased as well. What has changed is that minor violence on the part of girls, behavior that would not have been criminalized in the past, is now more likely to be viewed by teachers, police, and others as serious and threatening. Second, the stereotype of the passivity of women and girls has for too long been accepted. Now that greater attention is paid to intimate partner violence, girls naturally appear to be more violent than in the past (Mikel Brown et al., 2007). Finally, when looking at specific behaviors, girls more often perpetrate behaviors such as pushing, slapping, or biting, while boys are more likely to perpetrate in ways that are seriously harmful, such as punching or using a weapon as a threat (Whitaker et al., 2007). Furthermore, the etiology and meaning of intimate partner aggression may be quite different for girls versus boys (see Reed, Raj, Miller, & Silverman, 2010). The trend toward framing intimate partner violence among adolescents as gender neutral rather than embedded within gender-based historic, social, and political inequalities may serve to obscure rather than illuminate true understanding of intimate partner violence among adolescent girls with a concomitant danger of developing interventions and policy recommendations that are inadequate at best and harmful to girls at worst (Reed et al., 2010).

INTIMATE PARTNER VIOLENCE THEORIES

Feminist Theory

The feminist theory states that intimate partner violence is one form of an overarching phenomenon of male violence against women. Although usually applied in reference to adult intimate partner violence, the theory has implications for teen female dating violence. The theory postulates that male violence toward women is rooted in patriarchal social structures and in the cultural roles of men and women and is used to maintain subordinate social control and political status (Harway & O'Neill, 1999). Feminist theory focuses on the institutions and culture of a society instead of on individual physical strength or biological instinct to explain male violence against women (Harway & O'Neil, 1999). While feminist theory is used to explain heterosexual intimate partner violence perpetrated by men, the theory does not explain intimate partner violence in homosexual relationships or when females are the perpetrators.

Feminist theory focuses on patriarchal values that are learned and reinforced in most societies through gender role socialization, which establishes a belief in male entitlement, privilege, and domination. Patriarchal values are transferred to young males through intergenerational transmissions or through a society's institutions, such as the legal system, mass media, and the educational system (Harway & O'Neil, 1999). When a society's institutions are male dominated, the practices and policies reinforce patriarchal values and allow them to be legitimized and to flourish (Yodanis, 2004).

These patriarchal values may encourage young male teens to expect inequitable power relationships with females. One option used to maintain control and exert power for males is intimate partner violence (Yodanis, 2004). Intimate partner violence can include coercion, threats, intimidation, abuse, or force used by males to maintain control over females. Feminist theory implies that for an adolescent male to maintain control in an intimate relationship, the threat of violence can be as effective as actual physical violence (Harway & O'Neil, 1999).

Social Learning Theory

Albert Bandura's (1971) social learning theory states that individuals learn behaviors by internalizing the behaviors modeled by their social network. These behaviors are reinforced when the individual mimics the behavior and then receives some direct or indirect positive feedback. When applied to intimate partner violence, social learning theory suggests that individuals learn maladaptive or aggressive conflict resolution tactics by internalizing behaviors witnessed in their family of origin and then using similar conflict resolution tactics in their own intimate relationships. In other words, adolescents who witness parental intimate partner violence or who experienced abuse as a child are more likely to use violence in their own dating relationships. O'Keefe (1998) found in a sample of 232 adolescents who reported exposure to high levels of interparental violence that

49% reported perpetrating dating violence, while 55% reported being a victim of dating violence. However, the relationship between family of origin violence and intimate partner violence is inconsistent in the literature, which suggests multiple pathways from family of origin violence to later perpetration or victimization of dating violence.

The exploration of how social learning theory applies to dating violence has resulted in an interesting refinement. The inclusion of the consideration of gender socialization to Bandura's original theory can help distinguish between some of the pathways from family of origin violence to later experiences of intimate partner violence and perhaps help us understand some of the inconsistencies in the literature. Gwartney-Gibbs, Stockard, and Bohmer (1987) suggest that gender plays an important role in this theory in that boys and girls are socialized differently. These early effects of socialized gender differences may lead to different pathways from family of origin violence to intimate partner violence among girls and boys, particularly when additional risk factors are included. O'Keefe (1998), for example, found that low socioeconomic status, exposure to community and school violence, and acceptance of violence were the risk factors that predicted perpetration of dating violence in males who also witnessed high levels of parent to parent violence. For females, exposure to community and school violence and experiencing child abuse predicted perpetration of dating violence in females who had witnessed high levels of parent-to-parent violence, while Sims, Dodd, and Tejeda (2008) found that severe family of origin abuse predicted later perpetration of dating violence better in males than in females. These studies highlight the variability in how family of origin violence is internalized and the differential effects that these early childhood experiences may have on later intimate relationships in girls versus boys.

Attachment Theory

Researchers have drawn from and extended Bowlby's (1973) attachment theory in infants and young children to explain intimate partner violence among adolescents and adults. Bowlby described three attachment styles used to explain the relationship between young children and their caretakers. The three attachment styles described by Bowlby were secure attachment, avoidant attachment, and anxious-ambivalent attachment and were distinguished by the behaviors the young children showed during separation from their caregiver. These attachment styles become internal working models that shape how an individual interacts with others. Attachment theorists have expanded on this theory (in the form of adult attachment theory) to explain dating violence by proposing that intimate partner violence is an extreme reaction to the perception that an intimate partner is unavailable or lacks commitment to the relationship (Mayseless, 1991).

Attachment theory implies that adult attachment styles are extensions of our attachment style to our caregivers and therefore are characterized by certain beliefs and behaviors in our intimate relationships (e.g., Collins, Cooper, Albino,

& Allard, 2002). Secure attachment in adulthood is characterized by trust in an intimate partner and belief that one is loved and cared for by the partner. Those who express secure attachment also have high expectations for their relationships, are comfortable with intimacy (Collins et al., 2002), and are less likely to use aggressive or violent conflict resolution tactics with intimate partners. Avoidant attachment in adulthood is characterized by an emphasis on self-reliance and an unwillingness to depend on others. Those who express an avoidant attachment style view intimate partners as unreliable and are uncomfortable with intimacy (Collins et al., 2002; Mayseless, 1991). Adults with avoidant attachment may use passive-aggressive conflict resolution tactics such as disrespect, indifference, hostility, and contempt to distance themselves from an intimate partner. In contrast, individuals with an anxious-ambivalent attachment style in adulthood are characterized by an exaggerated need for closeness and intimacy. They may be unsure of the trustworthiness of their partner or may excessively worry about rejection (Collins et al., 2002), and these beliefs may lead to more aggressive responses to perceived inconsistency in their intimate partner (Mayseless, 1991). Attachment theorists suggest that intimate partner violence is more likely to occur when one or both partners have an insecure attachment style (avoidant or anxious-ambivalent). Those who express insecure attachment styles are characterized by uncertainty about the availability and responsiveness of their intimate partner when a threat to the relationship is perceived. Paired with poor conflict resolution tactics, this uncertainty may lead to violence as a tool to keep the partner in the relationship or to distance oneself from an intimate partner (Mayseless, 1991).

Socioecological Model

Bronfenbrenner's (1979) ecological theory states that the healthy development of an individual is dependent on the interconnections between several levels of a person's social world. Bronfenbrenner's theory speculates that there are complex layers of environment, each of which affects an individual's development and consequently that person's behavior. These levels can include individual, family, and community factors (1979). The interaction between factors in the model, such as personality, immediate family, and school/peer environment, and the larger community environment determines social and behavioral outcomes. Because these layers can interact with one another, researchers must look at not only each of the levels of influence but also the mechanisms that underlie their interactions.

Banyard, Cross, and Modecki (2006, p. 1315) described the interconnections of these micro and macro levels as "a series of concentric circles of influence, which include intrapersonal, family, peer, community, and wider societal influences on behavior and development." Dutton (2006) described Bronfenbrenner's (1979) theory as a nested ecological theory to highlight the importance of the interplay between a person's micro and macro influences on their development. This theory explains dating violence as a multicausal phenomenon, such that it is the presence of multiple predictors in different areas of a person's social world that influences the likelihood of aggressive behavior in an intimate relationship. Individual factors (e.g., low anger control, acceptance of violence), family factors (e.g., authoritarian parenting, low parental monitoring, parental conflict), peer factors (e.g., peer norms, peers' involvement in delinquency), and community factors (e.g., exposure to community violence, alienation in school) have all been linked to dating violence in adolescents. The interplay among these factors creates an environment that may lead to the use of violence in dating relationships. The socioecological model lends itself well to research that explores different correlates, predictors, risk, and protective factors simultaneously. Statistical methods that model complex relationships (i.e., structural equation models) are ideal for exploring the phenomenon of dating violence among adolescents from this perspective.

RISK AND PROTECTIVE FACTORS

One important step for understanding dating violence is to understand the risk factors that put adolescent girls at higher risk for involvement in dating violence. Research has identified multiple risk factors in females. Vezina and Hebert (2007) conducted a meta-analysis reviewing research that identified risk factors for psychological, physical, and sexual dating violence in adolescent females. Their meta-analysis grouped the risk factors into four categories that represent an ecological approach. The four categories of risk factors are sociodemographic factors, individual factors, environmental factors, and contextual factors.

Sociodemographic factors include age, ethnicity, socioeconomic status, family structure, type of living area, and religious practices (Vezina & Hebert, 2007). Age was inconsistently found to be a risk factor. The studies that found a relationship between age and dating violence found that older girls are more likely to be victims of dating violence (Halpern, Oslak, Young, Martin, & Kupper, 2001; Kreiter et al., 1999; Roberts, Klein, & Fisher, 2003; Silverman et al., 2001). Hokoda, Martin del Campo, and Ulloa (2011) found that 7th-grade adolescents report lower perpetration and victimization of verbal emotional abuse and jealous dating behaviors than 9th and 11th graders.

Research looking at ethnicity has also delivered inconsistent results. The research that has found a link between ethnicity and dating violence appears to support two different patterns. Some research has found that African American, Hispanic, and Asian American girls, compared to Caucasian girls, are at higher risk for victimization (Howard & Wang, 2003, 2005; Rickert, Wiemann, Harrykissoon, Berenson, & Kolb, 2002; Silverman et al., 2001), while other research has found that African American and Asian American girls are less likely to experience dating violence (Gover, 2004; Malik et al., 1997; O'Keefe & Treister, 1998; Silverman et al., 2001). Socioeconomic status as measured by parent's level of education or employment status, family income, or as a composite score of these factors, was not found to be associated with dating violence in 15 of the 20 studies looking at socioeconomic status. The 5 studies that did report a link between dating violence and socioeconomic status found a link between parent's level of education and dating violence. However, 3 studies found a positive association, while 2 studies found a negative association (Halpern et al., 2001; Magdol, Moffitt, Caspi, Newman, Fagan, & Silva, 1997; Magdol, Moffitt, Caspi, & Silva, 1998; Malik et al., 1997). Research indicates that the association between family structure and dating violence is more consistent in that not living with an intact family is a risk factor for dating violence (Billingham & Notebaert, 1993; Halpern et al., 2001; Magdol et al., 1998; Symons, Groer, Kepler-Youngblood, & Slater, 1994). Magdol et al. (1998) also identified living with both parents in adolescence as a protective factor against psychological dating violence in adulthood. Living in a rural area has also been found to be a risk factor for dating violence when compared to urban or suburban areas (Reuterman & Burcky, 1989; Spencer & Bryant, 2000). Vezina and Hebert (2007) found that 6 of the 10 studies considering religious practices as risk factors for dating violence found no link between the two. The 4 studies that did find a link between religious practices and dating violence found that girls who report no religious affiliations are at risk for sexual dating violence, while girls who do not consider religion important are at risk for psychological dating violence (Halpern et al., 2001; Maxwell, Robinson, & Post, 2003). In addition, Gover (2004) and Howard, Qiu, and Boekeloo (2003) found that participating in regular religious activities served as a protective factor against dating violence.

Individual factors as defined by Vezina and Hebert (2007) are internalizing problems, attitudes and beliefs about romantic relationships and sexuality, the presence of externalizing problems, romantic and sexual experiences, and school adaptation. Internalizing problems can be defined as depressive symptoms, suicidal behaviors, and low self-esteem. Depression was found to be associated with physical and sexual dating violence (Howard & Wang, 2003, 2005; Magdol et al., 1997; Vicary, Klingaman, & Harkness, 1995), while both depression and suicidal behavior were found to be both precursors and consequences of dating violence (Roberts et al., 2003). The link between self-esteem and dating violence is less clear, with some studies reporting an association between low self-esteem and dating violence, but longitudinal studies show no association between low self-esteem and dating violence (Cleveland, Herrera, & Stuewig, 2003; Follingstad, Rutledge, McNeill-Harkins, & Polek, 1992; Foshee, Benefield, Ennett, Bauman, & Suchindran, 2004; Jezl, Molidor, & Wright, 1996; O'Keefe, 1998; O'Keefe & Treister, 1998; Pirog-Good, 1992; Sharpe & Taylor, 1999; Small & Kerns, 1993). Research has not found a clear link between attitudes and beliefs about romantic relationships and sexuality. Research has looked at acceptance of dating violence, belief in the rape myth, an androcentric view of romantic and sexual relationships, and holding traditional gender stereotypes as risk factors; of these, acceptance of dating violence has been linked to dating violence in several studies (Clarey, Hokoda, & Ulloa, 2010; Malik et al., 1997; Muehlenhard & Linton, 1987; O'Keefe & Treister, 1998; Riggs & O'Leary, 1996). In addition, individual factors such as anger control beliefs and positive conflict resolution skills that include peaceful negotiation and compromise negatively relate to perpetration of dating violence (Antônio & Hokoda, 2009; Clarey et al., 2010; Feldman & Gowen, 1998; Wolf & Foshee, 2003; Wolfe, Scott, Reitzel-Jaffe, et al., 2001).

Research has shown that there is an association between dating violence and delinquent and antisocial behavior. Roberts et al. (2003) found that antisocial behaviors are both a precursor and a consequence of dating violence. With respect to girls, Ehrensaft, Cohen, Brown, Smailes, Chen, and Johnson (2003) and Magdol et al. (1998) found that women who reported more behavior problems as children and adolescents were at a higher risk for dating violence, although this relationship was mediated by family problems in childhood in the Ehrensaft et al. (2003) study. Drug and alcohol use in most studies has been linked to dating violence. Several studies found that substance abuse during a date is linked to sexual and physical violence (Howard & Wang, 2005; Kreiter et al., 1999; Muehlenhard & Linton, 1987; Synovitz & Byrne, 1998), while Cleveland et al. (2003) showed that alcohol consumption was associated with sexual victimization for casual dating partners but not for serious dating partners. Romantic and sexual promiscuity is linked to dating violence, such that the younger a girl is when she starts to have sex and the higher the number of sexual partners a girl has, her risk of being a victim of dating violence increases (Krahe, 1998; O'Keefe & Treister, 1998; Synovitz & Byrne, 1998; Vicary et al., 1995). Research has also found that not effectively using contraceptives is also a risk factor for dating violence. Along with ineffective use of contraceptives, teen pregnancy is a risk factor for physical and psychological dating violence (Howard & Wang, 2003, 2005; Kreiter et al., 1999; Rickert, Wiemann, et al., 2002). Prior victimization in dating relationships has also consistently been shown to be a risk factor for dating violence. Similarly, being a victim of one type of dating violence puts one at risk for other forms of dating violence (Himelein, 1995; Howard & Wang, 2005; Kreiter et al., 1999; Rickert, Wiemann, Vaughan, & White, 2004; Smith, White, & Holland, 2003). The last individual factor reviewed is school adaptation, and research has shown that girls who do not finish high school are at a greater risk for physical and psychological dating violence (Magdol et al., 1998; Maxwell et al., 2003; Reuterman & Burcky, 1989; Rickert, Wiemann, et al., 2002).

The third area of risk factors is environment factors. The environment factors reviewed are family variables and social network variables (Vezina & Hebert, 2007). Parental monitoring or the degree of parents' knowledge and supervision of their teens' behaviors predicts risky behaviors that include alcohol and drug use and dating violence. Straus and Savage (2005) report that neglectful behavior by parents is a consistent predictor of violence against dating partners across 17 nations. East, Chien, Adams, Hokoda, and Maier (2010) similarly report that mothers' monitoring of their daughter's whereabouts reduced their daughter's risk for dating violence victimization. In addition, having a sister who has been a victim of sexual abuse and dating violence is a risk factor for young women to have similar victimization experiences (East et al., 2010).

Other family variables include parental practices, witnessing family violence, and sexual abuse during childhood. Research has shown that harsh and punitive parenting, such as use of corporal punishment, is a risk factor for dating violence in every study that has looked at this type of parenting style (Ehrensaft et al., 2003; Magdol et al., 1998; Reuterman & Burcky, 1989; Small & Kerns, 1993). Girls who report not feeling close to their parents are at risk for dating violence when compared to girls who report being satisfied with how close they are to their parents (Cleveland et al., 2003; Ehrensaft et al., 2003; Magdol et al., 1998; Reuterman & Burcky, 1989). Witnessing family violence or being a victim of family violence was found to be a risk factor for dating violence in 19 of 26 studies (Arriaga & Foshee, 2004; Cyr, McDuff, & Wright, 2006; Ehrensaft et al., 2003; Follingstad et al., 1992; Foshee et al., 2004; Gagne, Lavoie, & Hebert, 2005; Hendy et al., 2003; Malik et al., 1997; Noland, Liller, McDermott, Coulter, & Seraphine, 2004; O'Keefe, 1998; O'Keeffe, Brockopp, & Chew, 1986; Reuterman & Burcky, 1989; Rosen, Bartle-Haring, & Stith, 2001; Sanders & Moore, 1999; Smith et al., 2003; Wekerle & Wolfe, 1998; Wekerle et al., 2001; Wolfe, Scott, Wekerle, & Pittman, 2001; Wolfe, Wekerle, Reitzel-Jaffe, & Lefebvre, 1998). Several studies have looked at the link between childhood sexual abuse and later dating violence victimization and have found a positive association between being a victim of childhood sexual abuse and dating violence victimization (Banyard, Arnold, & Smith, 2000; Cyr et al., 2006; Gagne et al., 2005; Himelein, Vogel, & Wachowiak, 1994; Sanders & Moore, 1999; Small & Kerns, 1993; Ulloa, Baerresen, & Hokoda, 2009). Cyr et al. (2006) found that specific factors regarding the sexual abuse, duration, presence of violence, and completion of intercourse increase the risk of dating violence victimization. Ulloa et al. (2009) found evidence that fear mediates the relationship between childhood sexual abuse and dating violence victimization.

Characteristics of an adolescent girl's peer groups can also put them at risk for dating violence. For example, knowing or having peers who have experienced dating violence, having peers who believe that dating violence is acceptable, and having delinquent peers put an adolescent girl at significant risk for dating violence (Arriaga & Foshee, 2004; Foshee et al., 2004; Reuterman & Burcky, 1989). The final environmental factor is exposure to community violence. Exposure to community violence has been linked to dating violence in that witnessing community violence and being a victim of community violence are risk factors for dating violence (Gagne et al., 2005; O'Keefe & Treister, 1998).

The final area of risk factors is the contextual factors associated with violence in dating relationships (Vezina & Hebert, 2007). Research has consistently shown that girls who date older men are at risk for physical and sexual dating violence (Buzy et al., 2004; Rickert et al., 2004). Other studies have found inconsistent contextual risk factors in the length and number of dating partners (Cleveland et al., 2003; Harned, 2002; Rickert et al., 2004). Studies have also reported a mutual nature to dating violence; a girl who is a perpetrator is also at risk for being a victim of dating violence (Cyr et al., 2006; Harned, 2002; Magdol et al., 1998; O'Keefe & Treister, 1998).

Vezina and Hebert's (2007) meta-analysis of risk factors for dating violence in adolescent females summarizes current research on dating violence risk factors. While their overview of risk factors helps to highlight what is currently known about risk factors, it also shows that there are areas where inconsistencies and gaps in knowledge exist. The risk factors that have been identified do not by themselves explain why some adolescent girls are involved in dating violence and others are not.

CONSEQUENCES OF INTIMATE PARTNER VIOLENCE AMONG ADOLESCENT GIRLS

In addition to the many risk factors that have been associated with adolescent dating violence victimization and perpetration, much work has been done in examining potential consequences of adolescent dating violence victimization. Many of the same physical and psychological health outcomes of dating violence and intimate partner violence identified among adult women have been shown to exist in adolescent female samples as well (Banyard & Cross, 2008). However, it is important to note that a major limitation of the majority of studies examining correlates of adolescent dating violence is that they are cross-sectional in design, and therefore causal associations or the establishment of temporal precedence cannot be made. Very few longitudinal studies of adolescent dating violence are able to examine mental and physical health correlates in a prospective manner (Ackard, Eisenberg, & Neumark-Sztainer, 2007; Chiodo, Wolfe, Crooks, Hughes, & Jaffe, 2009; Rich, Gidycz, Warkentin, Loh, & Weiland, 2005; Smith et al., 2003). Still, results from cross-sectional and longitudinal studies summarized below consistently indicate that adolescent dating violence is associated with a diverse set of psychological distress symptoms and other health concerns such as sexual risk behavior, substance use, and dating violence revictimization.

Mental Health Concerns

The majority of research on consequences of adolescent dating violence is in the area of mental health concerns such as depression, anxiety, and post-traumatic stress disorder (PTSD) symptoms (Ackard et al., 2007; Ackard, Neumark-Sztainer, & Hannan, 2003; Banyard & Cross, 2008; Callahan, Tolman, & Suanders, 2003; Wolitzky-Taylor et al., 2008); disordered eating and unhealthy weight control (Ackard & Neumark-Sztainer, 2002; Ackard et al., 2003; Rickert, Vaughan, & Wiemann, 2002; Silverman et al., 2001); and suicidal ideation and attempts (Ackard et al., 2003, 2007; Ackard & Neumark-Sztainer, 2002; Banyard & Cross, 2008; Olshen, McVeigh, Wunsch-Hitzig, & Rickert, 2007; Silverman et al., 2001). In addition, there has been research on the relationship between adolescent dating violence and other areas of health concern such as high-risk sexual behaviors and teen pregnancy among adolescent girls (Howard, Wang, & Yan, 2007; Silverman, Raj, & Clements, 2004; Silverman et al., 2001) and cigarette smoking and increased drug and alcohol use (Ackard et al., 2003, 2007; Ramisetty-Mikler, Goebert, Nishimura, & Caetano, 2006; Silverman et al., 2001). Research has also identified variables that may mediate the relationship between dating violence victimization and these mental health outcomes. For example, Filson, Ulloa, Runfola, and Hokoda (2010) report that feelings of relationship power explain the relationship between dating violence victimization and depression. Overall, the results from these studies presented above illustrate that adolescent dating violence can have a negative impact on the mental health of the adolescent girls who experience it and that additional public health policy, prevention, assessment, and interventions addressing adolescent dating violence are needed.

Revictimization

Another negative outcome of dating violence victimization is the potential for revictimization. A few longitudinal studies on dating violence among adolescents and college-age women have shown an association between dating violence victimization in adolescence (e.g., high school) and revictimization in college (Rich et al., 2005; Smith et al., 2003). The Rich et al. (2005) study both retrospectively and prospectively assessed physical dating violence among college women and found that having a history of physical dating violence victimization during adolescence predicted dating violence during the two-month follow-up period of the women. The Smith et al. (2003) study found that adolescence was the period during which young women were at greatest risk for physical dating violence and covictimization (defined as both physical and sexual assault occurring within the same time period but not necessarily simultaneously during a single violent event or with the same perpetrator), and young women who experienced physical dating violence victimization in high school were at significantly greater risk for physical dating violence victimization in college (revictimization). Results from these studies highlight the need to break the cycle between adolescent dating violence victimization and subsequent revictimization. The prevention of dating violence victimization during adolescence may also prevent dating violence victimization during college and adulthood. Smith et al. (2003, p. 1108) noted that "because young women who experience physical or sexual victimization in high school are at elevated risk for victimization in college, early intervention and treatment for these women is critical."

Educational Outcomes

Although not as extensive as the work on mental health consequences, there has been some research examining the relation between dating violence and educational outcomes among adolescents (Banyard & Cross, 2008), which is important given the centrality of school during this developmental period of life. Banyard and Cross (2008) examined mental health and educational consequences (school attachment, average grades, and thoughts of dropping out of school) of physical and sexual dating violence victimization in a convenience sample of adolescents in grades 7 to 12. Dating violence victimization was associated with poorer educational outcomes and higher levels of depression and suicidal thoughts. The results of this study support the idea for providing dating violence prevention efforts in schools, given the association between victimization and problems in mental health and school functioning.

SOCIAL SUPPORT

Despite the grave associations between adolescent dating violence, poor mental health, and other social and educational concerns, there is promising research on the buffering effects of social support. Holt and Espelage (2005) found that social support moderated the association between dating violence victimization and psychological well-being among African American and Caucasian adolescents. Likewise, Banyard and Cross (2008) found that greater perceived support was related to more positive outcomes among adolescents with histories of physical and sexual dating violence. Specifically, perceived parental and neighborhood support lowered suicidal thoughts for female sexual abuse victims compared with female nonvictims, and perceived neighborhood support also moderated the associations between physical abuse victimization and substance use and school attachment for adolescent girls (Banyard & Cross, 2008). Somewhat different from the other research, Salazar, Wingood, DiClemente, Lang, & Harrington (2004) found that social support was not a moderator but rather a mediator of the relation between dating violence victimization and psychological well-being among a group of African American adolescent girls. Further research is needed to examine the complex ways in which social support may affect the relationships between adolescent dating violence and negative outcomes. Nonetheless, research thus far highlights the potential importance of social connections as a coping resource for female adolescent victims of dating violence (Banyard & Cross, 2008).

INTERVENTION AND PREVENTION PROGRAMS

The research presented above demonstrates the prevalence and seriousness of intimate partner violence in teens and has described many risk and protective factors at different levels of influence. More work is needed to apply this research so that it informs the development of curriculum in prevention and intervention programs. Existing programs addressing teen dating violence have focused primarily on specific individual factors associated with violence, such as increasing knowledge about dating violence (e.g., Jaycox et al., 2006; Macgowan, 1997), and on addressing attitudes and norms by challenging acceptance of violence beliefs and gender stereotyping (e.g., Foshee & Langwick, 2004; Jaycox et al., 2006; Jones, 1998; Macgowan, 1997).

Fewer interventions have focused on building individual protective factors for teen dating violence. For example, more programs should focus on increasing anger management, social problem-solving skills, and positive conflict resolution skills (e.g., Foshee & Langwick, 2004), as research demonstrates that these individual skills negatively relate to perpetration of dating violence (e.g., Antônio &

Hokoda, 2009; Clarey et al., 2010; Feldman & Gowen, 1998; Wolf & Foshee, 2003). Particularly because youths admit that they are not confident in their ability to negotiate conflicts and have healthy dating relationships (Grover & Nangle, 2003; Lavoie, Robitaille, & Hebert, 2000; Sears, Byers, Whelan, & Saint-Pierre, 2006), prevention programs should increase efforts to teach these skills that may protect them from dating violence. Curricula that involve role-playing and modeling positive conflict resolution and anger control skills may be useful in programs (Burman, Margolin, & John, 1993; Cano et al., 1998). For example, individual skills that include positive communication, compromise, shared responsibility, self-regulation of arousal, and an ability to de-escalate conflict are all positive skills that should be promoted in prevention curricula. Support for this suggestion is also provided by research on adult couples that suggests that therapies that promote anger management and skills for de-escalating the intensity of conflicts may be effective for domestic violence characterized by reciprocal and bidirectional violence (e.g., Holtzworth-Munroe & Stuart, 1994; Holtzworth-Munroe, Meehan, Herron, Rehman, & Stuart, 2003; O'Leary & Smith Slep, 2006).

As our understanding of teen dating violence expands to include stalking behavior (Coker et al., 2008), relational aggression (Linder et al., 2002), and technologically advanced abuse (e.g., text messaging, social networking sites), curriculum development is needed to increase knowledge, challenge norms of acceptance, and teach coping skills and resources about these new types of abuse. Furthermore, interventions have only begun to address the range of individual factors linked to teen dating violence. In addition to addressing acceptance of violence beliefs, gender stereotyping (e.g., Foshee & Langwick, 2004; Jaycox et al., 2006), and anger management and social problem-solving skills (e.g., Foshee & Langwick, 2004), curricula could be developed to address other individual factors related to dating violence, such as anxious and avoidant attachment patterns. For example, addressing beliefs and behaviors that characterize anxious-ambivalent individuals, such as excessive worrying about rejection and jealous controlling behaviors (e.g., Collins et al., 2002), expands on interventions addressing teen relationship violence and is guided by attachment theory. Other individual factors, such as beliefs about relationship power inequities and one's proclivity for violence, could also be targeted in dating violence programs.

As research identifies more information about intimate partner violence in adolescents and its risk and protective factors from broader ecological levels of influence (e.g., family, peer, and cultural influences), these factors should be incorporated into curricula. There is a need for more prevention programs that target families of adolescents. Research that describes family factors such as authoritarian parenting, low parental monitoring, and sibling victimization (e.g., East et al., 2010; Simonelli, Mullis, Elliott, & Pierce, 2002; Straus and Savage, 2005) should be incorporated into parent education programs. Research suggests that addressing peer influence on dating violence is important (Schnurr & Lohman, 2008; Arriaga & Foshee, 2004; Brendgen, Vitaro, Tremblay, & Wanner, 2002). Furthermore, despite the need for culturally appropriate interventions for violence and other adolescent problems (Klevens, 2007; Le & Stockdale, 2008; Nation, 2003), few interventions address acculturative factors that may serve as risk and protective factors for teen dating violence in adolescents of color.

Prevention programs should address risk and protective factors for multiple problems across multiple social settings (Nation, 2003), yet most interventions addressing teen dating violence target only individual factors that include knowledge and normative beliefs about dating violence (Foshee & Reyes, 2009). Because substance abuse is linked to sexual and physical violence (e.g., Howard & Wang, 2005), programs should address these multiple problems together. Because younger age at first intercourse and higher number of sexual partners increases the risk of dating violence, which relates to higher incidences of teen pregnancy, addressing these multiple problems in a curriculum seems important.

Finally, researchers also recommend that prevention programs focus on specific developmental and situational challenges that youths face at different ages (Catalano & Hawkins, 1996). Nation (2003) also suggests that primary prevention programs should be offered when the topic (e.g., dating) is relevant to youths but before most youths have experienced the problem behavior (e.g., dating violence). Foshee and McNaughton Reyes (2009) suggest that this window is around 8th grade, or when teens are about 13 years old. Hokoda et al. (2007) report that dating violence increases between 7th and 9th grades, whereas other studies report that as many as a third of 6th-grade girls report dating violence victimization (Simon et al., 2010). The research suggests that prevention programs should start early, in late elementary school to early middle school. In addition, prevention programs should be adapted for the challenges common for specific age groups. For example, because college students are at risk for dating violence and binge drinking (Centers for Disease Control and Prevention, 2009; Wekerle & Wolfe, 1999) and are often facing additional stressors as they adjust to increased academic demands and living away from home, interventions should address these multiple problems (dating violence, alcohol abuse, academic and social stressors) in older adolescents in college.

REFERENCES

Ackard, D. M., Eisenberg, M. E., & Neumark-Sztainer, D. (2007). Long-term impact of adolescent dating violence on the behavioral and psychological health of male and female youth. *Journal of Pediatrics, 151*(5), 476–481. doi:10.1016/j.jpeds.2007.04.034

Ackard, D. M., & Neumark-Sztainer, D. (2002). Date violence and date rape among adolescents: Associations with disordered eating behavior and psychological health. *Child Abuse and Neglect, 26,* 455–473.

Ackard, D. M., Neumark-Sztainer, D., & Hannan, P. (2003). Dating violence among a nationally representative sample of adolescent girls and boys: Associations with behavioral and mental health. *Journal Of Gender-Specific Medicine: The Official Journal Of The Partnership for Women's Health at Columbia, 6*(3), 39–48.

Antônio, T., & Hokoda, A. (2009). Gender variations in dating violence and positive conflict resolution among Mexican adolescents. *Violence and Victims, 24*(4), 533–545. doi:10.1891/0886-6708.24.4.533

Arriaga, X. B., & Foshee, V. A. (2004). Adolescent dating violence: Do adolescents follow in their friends', or their parents', footsteps? *Journal of Interpersonal Violence, 19*(2), 162–184.

Baker, C. K., & Helm, S. (2010). Pacific youth and shifting thresholds: Understanding teen dating violence in Hawaii. *Journal of School Violence, 9,* 154–173.

Bandura, A. (1971). *Social learning theory.* New York: General Learning Press.

Banyard, V. L., Arnold, S., & Smith, J. (2000). Childhood sexual abuse and dating experiences of undergraduate women. *Child Maltreatment, 5*(1), 39–48.

Banyard, V. L., & Cross, C. (2008). Consequences of teen dating violence: Understanding intervening variables in ecological context. *Violence Against Women, 14*(9), 998–1013.

Banyard, V. L., Cross, C., & Modecki, K. L. (2006). Interpersonal violence in adolescence: Ecological correlates of self-reported perpetration. *Journal of Interpersonal Violence, 21*(10), 1314–1332.

Bennett, L., & Fineran, S. (1998). Sexual and severe physical violence among high school students: Power beliefs, gender, and relationship. *American Journal of Orthopsychiatry, 68,* 645–652.

Billingham, R. E. (1987). Courtship violence: The patterns of conflict resolution strategies across seven levels of emotional commitment. *Family Relations, 36*(3), 283.

Billingham, R. E., & Notebaert, N. L. (1993). Divorce and dating violence revisited: Multivariate analyses using Straus's conflict tactics subscores. *Psychological Reports, 73*(2), 679–684.

Bowlby, J. (1973). *Separation: Anxiety and Anger.* London: Hogarth.

Brendgen, M., Vitaro, F., Tremblay, R. E., & Wanner, B. (2002). Parent and peer effects on delinquency-related violence and dating violence: A test of two mediational models. *Social Development, 11*(2), 225–244.

Bronfenbrenner, U. (1979). *The ecology of human development experiments by nature and design.* Cambridge: Harvard University Press.

Burman, B., Margolin, G., & John, R. S. (1993). America's angriest home videos: Behavioral contingencies observed in home reenactments of marital conflict. *Journal of Consulting and Clinical Psychology, 61*(1), 28–39.

Buzy, W. M., McDonald, R., Jouriles, E. N., Swank, P. R., Rosenfield, D., Shimek, J. S., & Corbitt-Shindler, D. (2004). Adolescent girls' alcohol use as a risk factor for relationship violence. *Journal of Research on Adolescence, 14*(4), 449–470. doi:10.1111/j.1532-7795.2004.00082.x

Callahan, M. R., Tolman, R. M., & Saunders, D. G. (2003). Adolescent dating violence victimization and psychological well-being. *Journal of Adolescent Research, 18*(6), 664–681.

Cano, A., Avery-Leaf, S., Cascardi, M., & O'Leary, K. D. (1998). Dating violence in two high schools: Discriminating variables. *Journal of Primary Prevention, 18,* 431–446.

Cascardi, M., & Vivian, D. (1995). Context for specific episodes of marital violence: Gender and severity of violence differences. *Journal of Family Violence, 10*(3), 265–293. doi:10.1007/bf02110993

Catalano, S. (2007, December). Intimate partner violence in the United States. *National Crime Victimization Survey, Bureau of Justice Statistics.* Retrieved from www.ojp.usdoj.gov/bjs/.

Catalano, R. F., & Hawkins, J. D. (Eds.). (1996). *Social development model: A theory of antisocial behavior.* New York: Cambridge University Press.

Centers for Disease Control and Prevention. (n.d.). Intimate partner violence: Definitions. Retrieved on August 2, 2010, from http://www.cdc.gov/ViolencePrevention/intimatepartnerviolence/definitions.html.

Centers for Disease Control and Prevention. (2008, June 6). Youth Risk Behavior Surveillance: United States, 2007. *MMWR, 57,*(SS-4). Retrieved on June 21, 2011, from http://www.cdc.gov/mmwr/pdf/ss/ss5704.pdf.

Centers for Disease Control and Prevention. (2009). Understanding teen dating violence: Fact sheet. Retrieved on August 2, 2010, from http://www.cdc.gov/violenceprevention/pdf/TeenDatingViolence2009-a.pdf.

Chiodo, D., Wolfe, D. A., Crooks, C., Hughes, R., & Jaffe, P. (2009). Impact of sexual harassment victimization by peers on subsequent adolescent victimization and adjustment: A longitudinal study. *Journal of Adolescent Health, 45*(3), 246–252. doi:10.1016/j.jadohealth.2009.01.006

Clarey, A., Hokoda, A., & Ulloa, E. C. (2010). Anger control and acceptance of violence as mediators in the relationship between exposure to interparental conflict and dating violence perpetration in Mexican adolescents. *Journal of Family Violence, 25,* 619–625.

Cleveland, H. H., Herrera, V. M., & Stuewig, J. (2003). Abusive males and abused females in adolescent relationships: Risk factor similarity and dissimilarity and the role of relationship seriousness. *Journal of Family Violence, 18*(6), 325–339.

Coker, A. L., Sanderson, M., Cantu, E., Huerta, D., & Fadden, M. K. (2008). Frequency and types of partner violence among Mexican American college women. *Journal of American College Health, 56*(6), 665–673. doi:10.3200/jach.56.6.665-674

Collins, N. L., Cooper, M. L., Albino, A., & Allard, L. (2002). Psychosocial vulnerability from adolescence to adulthood: A prospective study of attachment style differences in relationship functioning and partner choice. *Journal of Personality, 70*(6), 965–1008.

Cyr, M., McDuff, P., & Wright, J. (2006). Prevalence and predictors of dating violence among adolescent female victims of child sexual abuse. *Journal of Interpersonal Violence, 21*(8), 1000–1017.

Dutton, D. G. (2006). *Rethinking domestic violence.* Vancouver: UBC Press.

Dutton, D. G., & Hemphill, K. J. (1992). Patterns of socially desirable responding among perpetrators and victims of wife assault. *Violence and Victims, 7,* 29–39.

East, P. L., Chien, N. C., Adams, J. A., Hokoda, A., & Maier, A. (2010). Links between sisters' sexual and dating victimization: The roles of neighborhood crime and parental controls. *Journal of Family Psychology, 24*(6), 698–708. doi:10.1037/a0021751

Ehrensaft, M. K., Cohen, P., Brown, J., Smailes, E., Chen, H., & Johnson, J. G. (2003). Intergenerational transmission of partner violence: A 20-year prospective study. *Journal of Consulting and Clinical Psychology, 71*(4), 741–753. doi:10.1037/0022-006x.71.4.741

Feldman, S. S., & Gowen, L. K. (1998). Conflict negotiation tactics in romantic relationships in high school students. *Journal of Youth and Adolescence, 27*(6), 691–717.

Filson, J., Ulloa, E., Runfola, C., & Hokoda, A. (2010). Does powerlessness explain the relationship between intimate partner violence and depression? *Journal of Interpersonal Violence, 25*(3), 400–415. doi:10.1177/0886260509334401

Follingstad, D. R., Rutledge, L. L., McNeill-Harkins, K., & Polek, D. S. (1992). Factors related to physical violence in dating relationships. In E. C. Viano (Ed.), *Intimate violence: Interdisciplinary perspectives* (pp. 121–135). Washington, DC: Hemisphere Publishing.

Foshee, V. A. (1996). Gender differences in adolescent dating abuse prevalence, types and injuries. *Health Education Research, 11,* 275–286.

Foshee, V. A., Benefield, T. S., Ennett, S. T., Bauman, K. E., & Suchindran, C. (2004). Longitudinal predictors of serious physical and sexual dating violence victimization during adolescence. *Preventive Medicine: An International Journal Devoted to Practice and Theory, 39*(5), 1007–1016. doi:10.1016/j.ypmed.2004.04.014

Foshee, V., & Langwick, S. (2004). *Safe dates: An adolescent dating abuse prevention curriculum.* Center City: Hazelden.

Foshee, V., & McNaughton Reyes, H. (2009). Primary prevention of adolescent dating abuse perpetration: When to begin, whom to target, and how to do it. In D. J. Whitaker & J. Lutzker (Eds.), *Preventing partner violence: Research and evidence-based intervention strategies* (pp. 141–168). Washington, DC: American Psychological Association.

Foshee, V. A., & Matthew, R. A. (2007). Adolescent dating abuse perpetration: A review of findings, methodological limitations, and suggestions for future research. In D. J. Flannery, A. T. Vazsonyi, & I. D. Waldman (Eds.), *The Cambridge handbook of violent behavior and aggression* (pp. 441–449). New York: Cambridge University Press.

Foshee, V. A., & Reyes, H. L. M. (2009). Primary prevention of adolescent dating abuse perpetration: When to begin, whom to target, and how to do it. In D. J. Whitaker & J. R. Lutzker (Eds.), *Preventing partner violence: Research and evidence-based intervention strategies* (pp. 141–168). Washington, DC: American Psychological Association.

Fox, J. A., & Zawitz, M. W. (n.d.). Homicide trends in the U.S. Department of Justice, Bureau of Justice Statistics. Retrieved on September 2, 2010, from http://bjs.ojp.usdoj.gov/content/homicide/intimates.cfm.

Freedner, N., Freed, L. H., Yang, Y. W., & Austin, S. B. (2002). Dating violence among gay, lesbian, and bisexual adolescents: Results from a community survey. *Journal of Adolescent Health, 31,* 469–474.

Gaertner, L., & Foshee, V. (1999). Commitment and the perpetration of relationship violence. *Personal Relationships, 6,* 227–239.

Gagne, M.-H., Lavoie, F., & Hebert, M. (2005). Victimization during childhood and revictimization in dating relationships in adolescent girls. *Child Abuse & Neglect, 29*(10), 1155–1172.

Gover, A. R. (2004). Childhood sexual abuse, gender, and depression among incarcerated youth. *International Journal of Offender Therapy and Comparative Criminology, 48*(6), 683–696. doi:10.1177/0306624x04264459

Gray, H. M., & Foshee, V. (1997). Adolescent dating violence: Differences between one-sided and mutually violent profiles. *Journal of Interpersonal Violence, 21,* 126–141.

Grover, R. L., & Nangle, D. W. (2003). Adolescent perceptions of problematic heterosocial situations: A focus group study. *Journal of Youth and Adolescence, 32*(2), 129–139. doi:10.1023/a:1021809918392

Gwartney-Gibbs, P. A., Stockard, J., & Bohmer, S. (1987). Learning courtship aggression: The influence of parents, peers, and personal experiences. *Family Relations, 36*(3), 276–282.

Halpern, C. T., Oslak, S. G., Young, M. L., Martin, S. L., & Kupper, L. L. (2001). Partner violence among adolescents in opposite-sex romantic relationships: Findings from the National Longitudinal Study of Adolescent Health. *American Journal of Public Health, 91*(10), 1679–1685.

Harned, M. S. (2002). A multivariate analysis of risk markers for dating violence victimization. *Journal of Interpersonal Violence, 17*(11), 1179–1197. doi:10.1177/088626002237401

Harway, M., & O'Neil, J. M. (Eds.). (1999). *What causes men's violence agianst women.* Thousand Oaks, CA: Sage.

Hendy, H. M., Weiner, K., Bakerofskie, J., Eggen, D., Gustitus, C., & McLeod, K. C. (2003). Comparison of six models for violent romantic relationships in college men and women. *Journal of Interpersonal Violence, 18*(6), 645–665. doi:10.1177/0886260503251180

Henton, J., Cate, R., Koval, J., Lloyd, S., & Christopher, S. (1983). Romance and violence in dating relationships. *Journal of Family Issues, 4*(3), 467–482. doi:10.1177/019251383004003004

Hickman, L. J., Jaycox, L. H., & Aronoff, J. (2004). Dating violence among adolescents: Prevalence, gender distribution, and prevention program effectiveness. *Trauma, Violence, & Abuse, 5,* 123–142.

Himelein, M. J. (1995). Risk factors for sexual victimization in dating: A longitudinal study of college women. *Psychology of Women Quarterly, 19*(1), 31–48. doi:10.1111/j.1471-6402.1995.tb00277.x

Himelein, M. J., Vogel, R. E., & Wachowiak, D. G. (1994). Nonconsensual sexual experiences in precollege women: Prevalence and risk factors. *Journal of Counseling & Development, 72*(4), 411–415.

Hokoda, A., Galvan, D. B., Malcarne, V. L., Castañeda, D. M., & Ulloa, E. C. (2007). An exploratory study examining teen dating violence, acculturation and acculturative stress in Mexican American adolescents. *Journal of Aggression, Maltreatment, & Trauma, 14,* 33–49.

Hokoda, A., Martin del Campo, M. A., & Ulloa E. C. (2011). *Age and gender differences in teen relationship violence.* Unpublished manuscript.

Holt, M. K., & Espelage, D. L. (2005). Social support as a moderator between dating violence victimization and depression/anxiety among African American and Caucasian adolescents. *School Psychology Review, 34*(3), 309–328.

Holtzworth-Munroe, A., Meehan, J. C., Herron, K., Rehman, U., & Stuart, G. L. (2003). Do subtypes of maritally violent men continue to differ over time? *Journal of Consulting and Clinical Psychology, 71*(4), 728–740.

Holtzworth-Munroe, A., & Stuart, G. L. (1994). Typologies of male batterers: Three subtypes and the differences among them. *Psychological Bulletin, 116,* 476–497. doi:10.1037/0033-2909.116.3.476

Howard, D. E., Qiu, Y., & Boekeloo, B. (2003). Personal and social contextual correlates of adolescent dating violence. *Journal of Adolescent Health, 33*(1), 9–17.

Howard, D. E., & Qi Wang, M. (2003). Risk procedures of adolescent girls who were victims of dating violence. *Adolescence, 38*(149), 1–14.

Howard, D. E., & Wang, M. Q. (2005). Psychosocial correlates of U.S. adolescents who report a history of forced sexual intercourse. *Journal of Adolescent Health, 36*(5), 372–379.

Howard, D. E., Wang, M. Q., & Yan, F. (2007). Prevalence and psychosocial correlates of forced sexual intercourse among U.S. high school adolescents. *Adolescence, 42*(168), 629–643.

Jaycox, L. H., McCaffrey, D., Eiseman, B., Aronoff, J., Shelley, G. A., Collins, R. L., & Marshall, G. N. (2006). Impact of a school-based dating violence prevention program among Latino teens: Randomized controlled effectiveness trial. *Journal of Adolescent Health, 39*(5), 694–704.

Jezl, D. R., Molidor, C. E., & Wright, T. L. (1996). Physical, sexual and psychological abuse in high school dating relationships: Prevalence rates and self-esteem issues. *Child & Adolescent Social Work Journal, 13*(1), 69–87.

Jones, L. (1998). The Minnesota School Curriculum Project: A statewide domestic violence prevention project in secondary schools. In B. Levy (Ed.), *Dating violence: Young women in danger* (pp. 258–266). Seattle, WA: Seal.
Kelly, P. J., Cheng, A.-L., Peralez-Dieckmann, E., & Martinez, E. (2009). Dating violence and girls in the juvenile justice system. *Interpersonal Violence, 24,* 1536–1551.
Klevens, J. (2007). An overview of intimate partner violence among Latinos. *Violence Against Women, 13*(2), 111–122. doi:10.1177/1077801206296979
Krahe, B. (1998). Sexual aggression among adolescents: Prevalence and predictors in a German sample. *Psychology of Women Quarterly, 22*(4), 537–554.
Kreiter, S. R., Krowchuk, D. P., Woods, C. R., Sinal, S. H., Lawless, M. R., & DuRant, R. H. (1999). Gender differences in risk behaviors among adolescents who experience date fighting. *Pediatrics, 104*(6), 1286–1292.
Lavoie, F., Robitaille, L., & Hebert, M. (2000). Teen dating relationships and aggression. *Violence Against Women, 6*(1), 6–36. doi:10.1177/10778010022181688
Le, T. N., & Stockdale, G. (2008). Acculturative dissonance, ethnic identity, and youth violence. *Cultural Diversity and Ethnic Minority Psychology, 14*(1), 1–9. doi:10.1037/1099-9809.14.1.1
Lewis, S. F., & Fremouw, W. (2001). Dating violence: A critical review of the literature. *Clinical Psychology Review, 21,* 105–127.
Linder, J. R., Crick, N. R., & Collins, W. A. (2002). Relational aggression and victimization in young adults' romantic relationships: Associations with perceptions of parent, peer, and romantic relationship quality. *Social Development, 11,* 69–86.
Macgowan, M. J. (1997). An evaluation of a dating violence prevention program for middle school students. *Violence and Victims, 12*(3), 223–235.
Magdol, L., Moffitt, T. E., Caspi, A., Newman, D. L., Fagan, J., & Silva, P. A. (1997). Gender differences in partner violence in a birth cohort of 21-year-olds: Bridging the gap between clinical and epidemiological approaches. *Journal of Consulting and Clinical Psychology, 65*(1), 68–78.
Magdol, L., Moffitt, T. E., Caspi, A., & Silva, P. A. (1998). Developmental antecedents of partner abuse: A prospective-longitudinal study. *Journal of Abnormal Psychology, 107*(3), 375–389. doi:10.1037/0021-843x.107.3.375
Malik, S., Sorenson, S. B., & Aneshensel, C. S. (1997). Community and dating violence among adolescents: Perpetration and victimization. *Journal of Adolescent Health, 21,* 291–302.
Marquart, B. S., Nannini, D. K., Edwards, R. W., Stanley, L. R., & Wayman, J. C. (2007). Prevalence of dating violence and victimization: Regional and gender differences. *Adolescence, 42,* 645–657.
Maxwell, C. D., Robinson, A. L., & Post, L. A. (2003). The nature and predictors of sexual victimization and offending among adolescents. *Journal of Youth and Adolescence, 32*(6), 465–477. doi:10.1023/a:1025942503285
Mayseless, O. (1991). Adult attachment patterns and courtship violence. *Family Relations, 40*(1), 21–28.
Mikel Brown, L., Chesney-Lind, M., & Stein, N. (2007). Patriarchy matters: Toward a gendered theory of teen violence and victimization. *Violence Against Women, 13,* 1249–1273.
Muehlenhard, C. L., & Linton, M. A. (1987). Date rape and sexual aggression in dating situations: Incidence and risk factors. *Journal of Counseling Psychology, 34*(2), 186–196.
Muñoz-Rivas, M. J., Graña, J. L., O'Leary, K. D., & González, M. P. (2007). Aggression in adolescent dating relationships: Prevalence, justification, and health consequences. *Journal of Adolescent Health, 40,* 298–304.

Nation, T. (2003). Creating a culture of peaceful school communities. *International Journal for the Advancement of Counselling, 25*(4), 309–315. doi:10.1023/b:adco.0000005530.72520.40

National Youth Risk Behavior Study. (2009). *YRBSS: Youth Risk Behavior Surveillance System.* Retrieved on October 1, 2010, from http://www.cdc.gov/healthyyouth/yrbs/index.htm.

Noland, V. J., Liller, K. D., McDermott, R. J., Coulter, M. L., & Seraphine, A. E. (2004). Is adolescent sibling violence a precursor to college dating violence? *American Journal of Health Behavior, 28,* S13.

O'Keefe, M. (1998). Factors mediating the link between witnessing interparental violence and dating violence. *Journal of Family Violence, 13*(1), 39–57.

O'Keefe, M., & Treister, L. (1998). Victims of dating violence among high school students: Are the predictors different for males and females? *Violence Against Women, 4*(2), 195–223.

O'Keeffe, N. K., Brockopp, K., & Chew, E. (1986). Teen dating violence. *Social Work, 31*(6), 465–468.

O'Leary, K. D., & Smith Slep, A. M. (2003). A dyadic longitudinal model of adolescent dating aggression. *Journal of Clinical Child and Adolescent Psychology, 32,* 314–327.

O'Leary, S. G., & Smith Slep, A. M. (2006). Precipitants of partner aggression. *Journal of Family Psychology, 20*(2), 344–347. doi:10.1037/0893-3200.20.2.344

O'Leary, K. D., Smith Slep, A. M., Avery-Leaf, S., & Cascardi, M. (2008). Gender differences in dating aggression among multiethnic high school students. *Journal of Adolescent Health, 42,* 473–479.

Olshen, E., McVeigh, K. H., Wunsch-Hitzig, R. A., & Rickert, V. I. (2007). Dating violence, sexual assault, and suicide attempts among urban teenagers. *Archives of Pediatrics & Adolescent Medicine, 161*(6), 539–545.

Ozer, E. J., Tschann, J. M., Pasch, L. A., & Flores, E. (2004). Violence perpetration across peer and partner relationships: Co-occurrence and longitudinal patterns among adolescents. *Journal of Adolescent Health, 34,* 67–71.

Pirog-Good, M. A. (1992). Sexual abuse in dating relationships. In E. C. Viano (Ed.), *Intimate violence: Interdisciplinary perspectives* (pp. 101–110). Washington, DC: Hemisphere Publishing.

Raiford, J. L., Wingood, G. M., & DiClemente, R. J. (2007). Prevalence, incidence, and predictors of dating violence: A longitudinal study of African American female adolescents. *Journal of Women's Health, 16,* 822–832.

Ramisetty-Mikler, S., Goebert, D., Nishimura, S., & Caetano, R. (2006). Dating violence victimization: Associated drinking and sexual risk behaviors of Asian, Native Hawaiian, and Caucasian high school students in Hawaii. *Journal of School Health, 76*(8), 423–429. doi:10.1111/j.1746-1561.2006.00136.x

Reed, E., Raj, A., Miller, E., & Silverman, J. G. (2010). Losing the "gender" in gender-based violence: The missteps of research on dating and intimate partner violence. *Violence Against Women, 16,* 348–354.

Renner, L., & Whitney, S. (2010). Examining symmetry in intimate partner violence among young adults using socio-demographic characteristics. *Journal of Family Violence, 25*(2), 91–106. doi:10.1007/s10896-009-9273-0

Reuterman, N. A., & Burcky, W. D. (1989). Dating violence in high school: A profile of the victims. *Psychology: A Journal of Human Behavior, 26*(4), 1–9.

Rich, C. L., Gidycz, C. A., Warkentin, J. B., Loh, C., & Weiland, P. (2005). Child and adolescent abuse and subsequent victimization: A prospective study. *Child Abuse & Neglect, 29*(12), 1373–1394.

Rickert, V. I., Vaughan, R. D., & Wiemann, C. M. (2002). Adolescent dating violence and date rape. *Current Opinion in Obstetrics and Gynecology, 14*(5), 495–500.

Rickert, V. I., Wiemann, C. M., Harrykissoon, S. D., Berenson, A. B., & Kolb, E. (2002). The relationship among demographics, reproductive characteristics, and intimate partner violence. *American Journal of Obstetrics and Gynecology, 187*(4), 1002–1007. doi:10.1067/mob.2002.126649

Rickert, V. I., Wiemann, C. M., Vaughan, R. D., & White, J. W. (2004). Rates and risk factors for sexual violence among an ethnically diverse sample of adolescents. *Archives of Pediatric & Adolescent Medicine, 158*(12), 1132–1139. doi:10.1001/archpedi.158.12.1132

Riggs, D. S., & O'Leary, K. D. (1996). Aggression between heterosexual dating partners. *Journal of Interpersonal Violence, 11*(4), 519–540. doi:10.1177/088626096011004005

Rivera-Rivera, L., Allen-Leigh, B., Rodríguez-Ortega, G., Chávez-Ayala, R., & Lazcano-Ponce, E. (2007). Prevalence and correlates of adolescent dating violence: Baseline study of a cohort of 7960 male and female Mexican public school students. *Preventive Medicine, 44*, 477–484.

Roberts, T. A., Klein, J. D., & Fisher, S. (2003). Longitudinal effect of intimate partner abuse on high-risk behavior among adolescents. *Archives of Pediatrics & Adolescent Medicine, 157*(9), 875–881. doi:10.1001/archpedi.157.9.875

Rosen, K. H., Bartle-Haring, S., & Stith, S. M. (2001). Using Bowen theory to enhance understanding of the intergenerational transmission of dating violence. *Journal of Family Issues, 22*(1), 124–142.

Salazar, L. F., Wingood, G. M., DiClemente, R. J., Lang, D. L., & Harrington, K. (2004). The role of social support in the psychological well-being of African American girls who experience dating violence victimization. *Violence and Victims, 19*(2), 171–187. doi:10.1891/vivi.19.2.171.64100

Sanders, B., & Moore, D. L. (1999). Childhood maltreatment and date rape. *Journal of Interpersonal Violence, 14*(2), 115–124. doi:10.1177/088626099014002001

Schnurr, M. P., & Lohman, B. J. (2008). How much does school matter? An examination of adolescent dating violence perpetration. *Journal of Youth and Adolescence, 37*(3), 266–283.

Sears, H. A., Byers, E. S., Whelan, J. J., & Saint-Pierre, M. (2006). "If it hurts you, then it is not a joke": Adolescents' ideas about girls' and boys' use and experience of abusive behavior in dating relationships. *Journal of Interpersonal Violence, 21*(9), 1191–1207.

Seligowski, A., & West, D. (2009). Aggression in dating relationships compared by country of origin. *College Student Journal, 43*, 1182–1190.

Sharpe, D., & Taylor, J. K. (1999). An examination of variables from a social-developmental model to explain physical and psychological dating violence. *Canadian Journal of Behavioural Science/Revue canadienne des Sciences du comportement, 31*(3), 165–175.

Silverman, J. G., Raj, A., & Clements, K. (2004). Dating violence and associated sexual risk and pregnancy among adolescent girls in the United States. *Pediatrics, 114*(2), e220–e225.

Silverman, J. G., Raj, A., Mucci, L. A., & Hathaway, J. E. (2001). Dating violence against adolescent girls and associated substance use, unhealthy weight control, sexual risk behavior, pregnancy, and suicidality. *JAMA, 286*, 572–579.

Simon, T. R., Miller, S., Gorman-Smith, D., Orpinas, P., & Sullivan, T. (2010). Physical dating violence norms and behavior among sixth-grade students from four U.S. sites. *Journal of Early Adolescence, 30*, 395–409.

Simonelli, C. J., Mullis, T., Elliott, A. N., & Pierce, T. W. (2002). Abuse by siblings and subsequent experiences of violence within the dating relationship. *Journal of Interpersonal Violence, 17*(2), 103–121.

Sims, E. N., Dodd, V. J. N., & Tejeda, M. J. (2008). The relationship between severity of violence in the home and dating violence. *Journal of Forensic Nursing, 4*(4), 166–173. doi:10.1111/j.1939-3938.2008.00028.x

Small, S. A., & Kerns, D. (1993). Unwanted sexual activity among peers during early and middle adolescence: Incidence and risk factors. *Journal of Marriage & the Family, 55*(4), 941–952. doi:10.2307/352774

Smith, P. H., White, J. W., & Holland, L. J. (2003). A longitudinal perspective on dating violence among adolescent and college-age women. *American Journal of Public Health, 93*(7), 1104–1109.

Spencer, G. A., & Bryant, S. A. (2000). Dating violence: A comparison of rural, suburban, and urban teens. *Journal of Adolescent Health, 27*(5), 302–305.

Straus, M. A. (1979). Measuring intrafamily conflict and violence: The Conflict Tactics (CT) Scales. *Journal of Marriage & the Family, 41*(1), 75–88.

Straus, M. A., & Savage, S. A. (2005). Neglectful behavior by parents in the life history of university students in 17 countries and its relation to violence against dating partners. *Child Maltreatment: Journal of the American Professional Society on the Abuse of Children, 10*(2), 124–135.

Symons, P. Y., Groer, M. W., Kepler-Youngblood, P., & Slater, V. (1994). Prevalence and predictors of adolescent dating violence. *Journal of Child and Adolescent Psychiatric Nursing, 7*(3), 14–23.

Synovitz, L. B., & Byrne, T. J. (1998). Antecedents of sexual victimization: Factors discriminating victims from nonvictims. *Journal of American College Health, 46*(4), 151.

Teten, A. L., Ball, B., Valle, L. A., Noonan, R., & Rosenbluth, B. (2009). Considerations for the definition, measurement, consequences, and prevention of dating violence victimization among adolescent girls. *Journal of Women's Health, 18,* 923–927.

Ulloa, E. C., Baerresen, K., & Hokoda, A. (2009). Fear as a mediator for the relationship between child sexual abuse and victimization of relationship violence. *Journal of Aggression, Maltreatment & Trauma, 18*(8), 872–885.

Vezina, J., & Hebert, M. (2007). Risk factors for victimization in romantic relationships of young women: A review of empirical studies and implications for prevention. *Trauma, Violence, & Abuse, 8*(1), 33–66. doi:10.1177/1524838006297029

Vicary, J. R., Klingaman, L. R., & Harkness, W. L. (1995). Risk factors associated with date rape and sexual assault of adolescent girls. *Journal of Adolescence, 18*(3), 289–306. doi:10.1006/jado.1995.1020

Wekerle, C., & Wolfe, D. A. (1998). The role of child maltreatment and attachment style in adolescent relationship violence. *Development and Psychopathology, 10*(3), 571–586.

Wekerle, C., & Wolfe, D. A. (1999). Dating violence in mid-adolescence: Theory, significance, and emerging prevention initiatives. *Clinical Psychology Review, 4,* 435–456.

Wekerle, C., Wolfe, D. A., Hawkins, D. L., Pittman, A.-L., Glickman, A., & Lovald, B. E. (2001). Childhood maltreatment, post-traumatic stress symptomatology, and adolescent dating violence: Considering the value of adolescent perceptions of abuse and a trauma mediational model. *Development and Psychopathology, 13*(4), 847–871.

Whitaker, D. J., Haileyesus, T., Swahn, M., & Saltzman, L. S. (2007). Differences in frequency of violence and reported injury between relationships with reciprocal and nonreciprocal intimate partner violence. *American Journal of Public Health, 97,* 941–947.

Wolf, K. A., & Foshee, V. A. (2003). Family violence, anger expression styles, and adolescent dating violence. *Journal of Family Violence, 18*(6), 309–316.

Wolfe, D. A., Scott, K., Reitzel-Jaffe, D., Wekerle, C., Grasley, C., & Straatman, A.-L. (2001). Development and validation of the Conflict in Adolescent Dating Relationships Inventory. *Psychological Assessment, 13*(2), 277–293.

Wolfe, D. A., Scott, K., Wekerle, C., & Pittman, A.-L. (2001). Child maltreatment: Risk of adjustment problems and dating violence in adolescence. *Journal of the American Academy of Child & Adolescent Psychiatry, 40*(3), 282–289.

Wolfe, D. A., Wekerle, C., Reitzel-Jaffe, D., & Lefebvre, L. (1998). Factors associated with abusive relationships among maltreated and nonmaltreated youth. *Developmental Psychopathology, 10*(1), 61–85.

Wolitzky-Taylor, K. B., Ruggiero, K. J., Danielson, C. K., Resnick, H. S., Hanson, R. F., Smith, D. W., Saunders, B. E., & Kilpatrick, D. G. (2008). Prevalence and correlates of dating violence in a national sample of adolescents. *American Academy of Child and Adolescent Psychiatry, 47,* 755–762.

Yodanis, C. L. (2004). Gender inequality, violence against women, and fear. *Journal of Interpersonal Violence, 19*(6), 655–675. doi:10.1177/0886260504263868

Chapter 10

A Feminist Identity Development Model for Filipina Americans

The Influences of Discrimination on Psychological Well-Being and Self-Esteem

Kevin L. Nadal

INTRODUCTION

Individuals who identify with more than one group are often asked to choose one identity over the other. Biracial people are often given one box to select on demographic forms and/or are asked questions about which parent they identify with more (Johnston & Nadal, 2010; Root, 1997), while lesbian, gay, bisexual, and transgender (LGBT) persons of color are often pressured to join either a general White LGBT community or be closeted in their respective racial/ethnic communities (Chan, 1989; Conerly, 1996). Existing literature in psychology and education tends to follow this trend, whereby social groups are studied in broader terms without examining how intersections of various cultural identities may impact individual experiences. For example, previous LGBT literature assumes a universal LGBT experience without accounting for variations of identity that may occur as a result of gender, race, ethnicity, religion, or social class (Nadal, Rivera, & Corpus, 2010). At the same time, studies of feminism tend to concentrate primarily on White women without understanding how being a woman of color can impact one's gender, feminist identity development, and/or experiences with sexism (Bowman et al., 2001). As a result, individuals who identify with any subgroup within a larger group may often feel invisible and marginalized.

One group that is often invisible is Filipino Americans. While Filipino Americans may be the second-largest Asian American group in the United States as well as the second-largest immigrant population in the United States, they are often lumped into a general Asian American category without being recognized for their unique social and cultural traits (Nadal, 2004, 2011). Filipinos have a distinctive colonial history resulting from Spanish colonialism for almost 400 years and American colonialism for 50 years. The Philippines is the only Asian country to be predominantly Roman Catholic and one of two Asian countries to have English as a national language. Filipino Americans are the only racial/ethnic group that has been categorized by the government in a multitude of ways (including Asian, Pacific Islander, and Hispanic). Filipino Americans are the only Asian group regularly mistaken as members of other racial/ethnic groups (e.g., Latino, Arab, multiracial), and Filipino Americans are the only Asian ethnicity to be recognized as a distinct category on the U.S. census apart from "Asian" or "Pacific Islander" (Nadal, 2004, 2011).

This invisibility for Filipino Americans becomes even more prominent because of the model minority myth, which stereotypes all Asian Americans as being model and compliant citizens who succeed academically and vocationally. While seemingly a compliment, Nadal and Sue (2009) cite many problems with this stereotype. First, because Asian Americans are assumed to be successful, it is common for there to be limited outreach, scholarship, or public assistance toward the group. For example, most scholarship programs for underrepresented racial minority groups tend to exclude Asian Americans and only include African Americans, Latinos, and Native Americans. Second, because Asian Americans are stereotyped as the model minority, these other aforementioned racial groups are viewed as the opposite of the model (i.e., criminals, intellectual inferiors, etc.), resulting in tension between these two groups. Finally, there are many Asian American ethnic groups that experience educational and health disparities that are contrary to the myth. For example, Southeast Asians tend to live in poverty more so than the general American population and the Asian American population (Reeves & Bennett, 2004). Consequently, many issues affecting these Asian American groups may be overlooked.

Filipino Americans maintain many of these sociocultural and educational experiences that are quite the opposite of the model minority. Filipino Americans have among the highest high school dropout and lowest college admission rates of all minority groups as well as the highest rates of teen and out-of-wedlock pregnancy and the highest reported incidents of HIV/AIDS out of all Asian American groups (Nadal, 2004, 2011). Because of the model minority myth, Filipino Americans (and other marginalized Asian American groups) continue to be unnoticed and neglected. Additionally, Filipino Americans are often viewed as not Asian enough or as the bottom of the Asian hierarchy by other Asian Americans because of their darker skin color and/or stereotypes of intellectual inferiority. Consequently, many Filipino Americans may choose to distinguish themselves as a unique ethnic group by celebrating an ethnocentric Filipino identity while rejecting an Asian American racial identity (Nadal, 2004, 2011).

Because Filipino Americans are invisible in the greater society, there has been a dearth in literature focusing on subgroups within the community. Much in the same way that literature assumes a universal Asian American experience regardless of ethnicity, the literature in psychology and education largely assumes a universal Filipino American experience. Research involving identity development, coping mechanisms, depression, and experiences with racism tends to highlight Filipinos as a general group without considering gender, sexual orientation, and other social identities. For example, while the Filipino American identity development model has been used by practitioners to better understand Filipino Americans, it focuses on Filipino Americans as a general population without examining differences that may occur as a result of gender or other social identities. Similarly, while identity development models have been used to understand gender (e.g., Downing & Roush, 1985) and sexual orientation (e.g., Troiden, 1989), they often fail to consider how race or ethnicity influence these processes.

The purpose of this chapter is to examine the identity development of Filipino American women, or Filipinas. By examining the intersections of two identity models—the Filipino American Identity Development Model (Nadal, 2004) and a feminist identity model (Downing & Roush, 1985)—one can understand how various social identities are directly related to each other. Furthermore, by examining intersectional identities, one can become aware of how one's worldviews and experiences may influence one's self-esteem and mental health. Finally, the chapter will investigate how discrimination (particularly racism and sexism) may influence Filipinas' psychological well-being in negative ways while sometimes pushing them to healthier identities.

PREVIOUS IDENTITY DEVELOPMENT MODELS

Filipino American Identity Development

The Filipino American Identity Development Model is a six-stage model that aims to serve as a framework for counselors and other practitioners in understanding the ethnic identity development of Filipino American clients (Nadal, 2004). In an updated version of the model, "stages" were renamed "statuses" to signify that individuals' experiences are more fluid. Through these six statuses, it is expected that practitioners may be conscious of the various worldviews of their clients in order to provide the most culturally competent services for them. Status 1, Ethnic Awareness, is when a child understands that she or he is Filipino, based on the people, traditions, languages, and foods that surround her or him. Because the child is surrounded mostly by her or his family, being Filipino would be the norm, resulting in positive or neutral feelings about other Filipinos. Status 2, Assimilation to Dominant Culture, is when an individual attempts to assimilate into the dominant culture by rejecting her or his cultural foods, accents, and anything that distinguishes her or him from Whites. As an individual enters school systems or is exposed to mainstream media, it may be likely for the individual to see that White American norms are dominant. As a result, Filipinos (and other people of color) may view their own values, traditions, and standards of beauty as inferior to Whites. Status 3, Social Political Awakening, is when the individual becomes actively aware of racism in society; this can be triggered by something negative (e.g., a racially discriminatory experience) or something positive (e.g., learning about one's family history). Individuals may react differently in this status; some may view all Whites as being bad or racist, while others may aim to maintain interpersonal and romantic relationships with only people of color.

The next two statuses of identity development differentiate the Filipino American Identity Development Model from other racial or ethnic identity development models. Status 4, Panethnic Asian American Consciousness, is a status in which the Filipino adopts an Asian American identity. In this status, individuals may feel a connection with other Asian American ethnic groups (e.g., East Asians, Southeast Asians, and South Asians) and develop an Asian American identity. Meanwhile, Status 5, Ethnocentric Realization, is a status in which the Filipino American may realize her or his marginalized role in the Asian American community and develop a pro-Filipino identity. This may be triggered by a discriminatory experience by an Asian American or by learning of the historically marginalized experience of Filipinos within the Asian American diaspora in an ethnic studies class. Finally, Status 6, Introspection, is a status in which the Filipino American is comfortable with her or his identity as a person of color while recognizing the costs and benefits of both panethnic and ethnocentric identities. The individual in this stage realizes how tiresome it is to fixate on race but finds other ways to remain committed to social justice.

Feminist Identity Development

Downing and Roush's (1985) proposed model of feminist identity development was created to demonstrate how women learn to achieve a positive feminist identity by accepting, grappling with, and processing their feelings about sexism and gender discrimination. It is a five-stage identity development model that highlights similar stages and individual progression as other racial identity development models. Stage 1, Passive Acceptance, is a stage in which a woman is oblivious to sexism, denies that individual or institutional sexism exists, or both. This status may be exemplified by a woman who allows men to treat her in mysogynistic ways, who denies that sexism impacts her everyday life, or who believes that men are superior intellectually or physically. Stage 2, Revelation, is when a woman becomes aware of sexism (e.g., through experiencing sexual harassment or studying sexism in a women's studies course). This stage usually leads to conflicting feelings of anger and guilt in which the woman wonders how she was ever blind to sexism. Stage 3, Embeddedness-Emanation, is when women may develop close emotional connections with other women and form a sisterhood or support system; women may turn to each other so they can feel affirmed in their new identities and feel validated with others who recognize sexism in the same ways that they do. Stage 4, Synthesis, is when an individual learns to value being a woman through transcending traditional sex roles and valuing men individually instead of stereotypically. Finally, Stage 5, Active Commitment, involves the translation of an integrated identity into one in which the woman is moved to meaningful and effective action.

Filipina American Feminist Identity Model

Because racial and ethnic experiences will influence one's identity development as a woman (and vice versa), it is important for practitioners to take both identities into consideration when working with their clients. However, as aforementioned, most identity development models tend to view a person's singular identities without recognizing how intersectional identities affect a person's psychological processes. Understanding intersectional identities is necessary for psychologists, counselors, educators, and other practitioners in order to provide the most culturally appropriate services for their clients. Thus, the Filipina American Feminist Identity Development Model is proposed in order for practitioners to be conscious of racial, ethnic, and feminist identity development with Filipina Americans. The model acknowledges the marginalization of women of color within the feminist movement in addition to the invisibility of Filipino Americans in general society. In addition, the model is a call to end the use of universal identities and to consider the influence of multiple salient identities that influence an individual at any given time. Table 10.1 outlines the varying statuses in which racial/ethnic and gender identities may intersect and result in a distinctive identity. Stages 4 and 5 in the Feminist Identity Model are combined into one stage, as the emotional processes, values, and characteristics that may be occurring in both have similar undertones. Meanwhile, Stage 1 from the Filipino American Identity Development Model is being withdrawn, as it is a stage that is proposed to occur in early childhood.

In reviewing Table 10.1, there are several identity statuses that would be beneficial to examine, as they may represent a spectrum of experiences for Filipina Americans. Status 1, Passive Acceptance Assimilation, occurs when an individual is unaware of or oblivious to her status as a woman and as a racial/ethnic minority. The woman in this status may have both internalized racism and sexism, whereby she does not like being Asian, Filipina, or a woman. A woman at this status may allow men to make sexist and/or racist jokes toward her and may even allow White men to exoticize her. Status 4, Passive Acceptance Ethnocentric Consciousness, is when a woman might only interact with other Filipino Americans but allows Filipino American men to take advantage of her and/or treat her as an inferior. Status 7, Revelation Sociopolitical Awakening, transpires when a woman might feel

Table 10.1
Filipina feminist identity model

	Assimilation	Sociopolitical Awakening	Panethnic Consciousness	Ethnocentric Consciousness	Integration
Passive Acceptance	Status 1: Low feminist ID, Low RI, Low EI	Status 2: Low feminist ID, Conflicted RI, Conflicted EI	Status 3: Low feminist ID, High RI, Neutral EI	Status 4: Low feminist ID, Low RI, High EI	Status 5: Low feminist ID, Integrated RI, Integrated EI
Revelation	Status 6: Conflicted feminist ID, Low RI, Low EI	Status 7: Conflicted feminist ID, Conflicted RI, Conflicted EI	Status 8: Conflicted feminist ID, High RI, Neutral EI	Status 9: Conflicted feminist ID, Low RI, High EI	Status 10: Conflicted feminist ID, Integrated RI, Integrated EI
Embeddedness/ Emanation	Status 11: High feminist ID, Low RI, Low EI	Status 12: High feminist ID, Conflicted RI, Conflicted EI	Status 13: High feminist ID, High RI, Neutral EI	Status 14: High feminist ID, Low RI, High EI	Status 15: High feminist ID, Integrated RI, Integrated EI
Synthesis/ Active Commitment	Status 16: Integrated feminist ID, Low RI, Low EI	Status 17: Integrated feminist ID, Conflicted RI, Conflicted EI	Status 18: Integrated feminist ID, High RI, Neutral EI	Status 19: Integrated feminist ID, Low RI, High EI	Status 20: Integrated feminist ID, Integrated RI, Integrated EI

- RI = Racial identity.
- EI = Ethnic identity.

conflicted as she learns about the sexism that she experiences as a woman while also realizing the racism that she experiences as a person of color. Statuses 13 and 14 represent instances in which a Filipina American may identify primarily with her Asian American identity or her Filipina American identity. For example, a woman in Status 13, Embeddedness/Emanation Panethnic Consciousness, may turn to a general community of Asian American women for support and solidarity, while a woman in Status 14, Embeddedness/Emanation Ethnocentric Consciousness, may require finding a support system of only other Filipina American women. Status 16, Synthesis/Active Commitment Assimilation, might represent a woman who is comfortable with her identity as a woman yet may reject her identity as a person of color. This woman may have other White feminist friends yet may not be concerned about issues impacting people of color. Status 20, Synthesis/Active Commitment Integration, represents an individual who is fulfilled as a Filipina, an Asian, a person of color, and a woman.

There are many ways that a person's identity development status may influence self-esteem and mental health. For example, if a Filipina American exhibits characteristics of assimilation or passive-acceptance, it may be possible that she has internalized racism or internalized sexism. These feelings of internalized oppression may have direct influences on her self-esteem and self-efficacy. Perhaps this low self-esteem may lead to mental health problems such as depression, anxiety, or body image issues. Perhaps this low self-efficacy can lead to her a lack of self-confidence, which may then impact her performance levels and her ability to achieve her goals. Conversely, if a Filipina American exhibits a more integrative or synthesized identity, she may have a higher self-esteem, which may serve as a protective factor for mental health problems. She may develop a self-confidence that may help her to achieve her goals while overcoming the potential racism and sexism that may prevent her from doing so.

Filipino Americans (both women and men) may also deal with a colonial mentality, which may also negatively impact identity development and mental health. Colonial mentality is defined as the denigration of a person's self and culture in which the mores of the colonizer are viewed as superior, while the mores of the indigenous or oppressed are viewed as inferior (David, 2008). Colonial mentality can manifest through a person's denigration of self or group, particularly through language or standard of beauty. For Filipinos specifically, colonial mentality involves the denigration of native and indigenous Filipino values while uplifting Spanish and American colonial values. Some Filipino Americans may denigrate all other Filipinos, while some may discriminate based on skin color, regional background, education, or language. For example, hierarchies in the Philippines (and the Filipino American community) in which those who are lighter-skinned are viewed as the most attractive or beautiful, and those who are darker-skinned are viewed as the least attractive. Filipino Americans who speak the most "proper" American English (i.e., without a noticeable Filipino accent) would be viewed as the most educated with the most leadership potential, while those who are FOBs (recent immigrants who are "fresh off the boat") are viewed as intellectually inferior, uncivilized, or out of date.

Previous research has found that colonial mentality is a significant predictor of depression (David, 2008). Hence, it is important for practitioners to be aware of their clients' levels of colonial mentality in order to promote optimal mental health. For women specifically, it is important to recognize how colonial mentality may impact both their racial and gender identities. Because of these colonial standards of beauty in the Philippines as well as the influence of the American media, Filipino Americans may be taught that unrealistic standards of beauty (e.g., lighter skin, being skinny, or having slender bodies) are the norm. Many Filipinas may take different measures to achieve these norms, including bleaching their skin, lightening their hair, or developing eating disorders. Perhaps if these women were taught to be proud of their racial or ethnic identities while being taught that they are beautiful at any size, some of these mental health problems could decrease in the community.

THE RELATIONSHIP BETWEEN DISCRIMINATION AND IDENTITY

In reviewing the Filipina American Feminist Identity Model, one may notice how racism, sexism, and the intersections of both influence a person's identity development. When a person of color experiences racism or when a woman experiences sexism, there are many ways that the individual may react. Some people may simply choose to ignore the acts, sometimes remaining oblivious to the various ways that oppression affects their everyday lives and their relationships. And as aforementioned, some of these individuals may internalize that they are somehow inferior or blameworthy, which potentially may lead to mental health issues such as low self-esteem, depression, or anxiety. On the other hand, when some people experience discrimination, they may become angered or frustrated, which may advance them to more socially conscious identities. Thus, while discriminatory experiences obviously have negative consequences, there are some positive reactions that may occur. In fact, in many ways, experiencing discrimination may be somewhat necessary in heightening one's social and political awareness.

At the same time, it appears that a person's identity can actually influence the individual's ability to recognize discrimination when it occurs, which may then impact the various ways that individuals react in such situations and how they cope with such negative experiences. In a study examining women's perceptions of gender microaggressions, or subtle forms of discrimination, women who appeared to have higher levels of feminist identity were much more able to identify sexist experiences when they occurred (Capodilupo et al., 2010). When women are able to recognize discrimination, particularly in more subtle forms, perhaps they are able to cope with such instances in healthier ways. For example, if a woman experiences a gender microaggression at work (e.g., a male coworker consistently makes subtle remarks about her body), there are many ways that she may react. A woman with a less developed feminist identity may not recognize that his behavior is inappropriate and sexist; thus, she may not confront him on his behavior, which then enables him to continue. As a result, it is possible that she may feel uncomfortable in coming to work, leading to greater tension and anxiety that may affect her work, her performance, or her mental health. Conversely, a woman with a more developed feminist identity may more easily comprehend the sexist nature of her male coworker's behavior, which may lead to more favorable responses. She may have the confidence to confront him on the situation or report his behavior to a supervisor or human resources personnel. She may choose not to challenge him but instead turn to other coworkers or friends for support or validation. Either way, she may have a better grasp of her emotional reactions, which may then assist her in selecting the most appropriate and beneficial coping mechanism.

Finally, it appears that the discrimination that a person experiences more (or that is more salient at the time) may influence that person's identities. If a Filipina American is consistently experiencing racism at work or school, she may be more attuned to racial dynamics, may have an easier time in identifying racist behaviors, and may hold on to a more Filipino identity than her feminist identity. On the contrary, if a Filipina American is constantly dealing with sexism in her family or other situations, her identity as a woman may be the most salient for her. In either of these cases, one identity may be heightened more than another. However, there are many instances when an individual is unclear about whether a discriminatory experience is occurring because of her race, her ethnicity, her gender, or some combination of all three. For example, if a 20-year-old Filipina American perceives a supervisor or other authority figure speaking with her in a more condescending tone, she may be confused as to whether the behavior is because of her identity as a woman, an Asian American, a Filipina, or a young person. In these types of instances, the ambiguous intentions behind the discrimination may strengthen an individual's intersectional identity; an individual may recognize that her experience as a woman of color or as a Filipina American cannot be separated. She cannot choose which identity is more salient to her because they are both salient, sometimes equally and sometimes not.

While this chapter presented the various identity statuses that Filipina Americans may experience throughout their lives, it is also crucial to recognize that there are other intersectional identities that can add complexities to this model even further. For example, lesbian and transgender women, working-class women, and disabled women may have additional dimensions of identity that may further complicate their experiences with discrimination and their identity development. Indeed, it appears that the more marginalized identities an individual experiences, the more complex her identity may be. Thus, it is essential for practitioners to continue to advocate for marginalized groups, particularly those with multiple oppressed identities, in order to ensure that everyone's voices are heard.

REFERENCES

Bowman, S. L., Rasheed, S., Ferris, J., Thompson, D. A., McRae, M., & Weitzman, L. (2001). Interface of feminism and multiculturalism: Where are the women of color? In J. Ponterotto, J. Casas, L. Suzuki, & C. Alexander (Eds.), *Handbook of multicultural counseling* (pp. 779–798). Thousand Oaks, CA: Sage.

Capodilupo, C. M., Nadal, K. L., Corman, L., Hamit, S., Lyons, O., & Weinberg, A. (2010). The manifestation of gender microaggressions. In D. W. Sue (Ed.), *Microaggressions and marginality: Manifestation, dynamics, and impact* (pp. 193–216). New York: Wiley.

Chan, C. (1989). Issues of identity development among Asian-American lesbians and gay men. *Journal of Counseling & Development, 68,* 16–20.

Conerly, G. (1996). The politics of Black, lesbian, gay, and bisexual identity. In B. Beemyn & M. Eliason (Eds.) *A lesbian, gay, bisexual, and transgender anthology* (pp. 133–145). New York: New York University Press.

David, E. J. R. (2008). A colonial mentality model of depression for Filipino Americans. *Cultural Diversity and Ethnic Minority Psychology, 14,* 118–127.

Downing, N. E., & Roush, K. L. (1985). From passive acceptance to active commitment: A model of feminist identity development for women. *Counseling Psychologist, 13,* 695–709.

Johnston, M. P., & Nadal, K. L. (2010). Multiracial microaggressions: Exposing monoracism in everyday life and clinical practice. In D. W. Sue (Ed.), *Microaggressions and marginality: Manifestation, dynamics, and impact* (pp. 123–144). New York: Wiley.

Nadal, K. L. (2004). Filipino American identity development model. *Journal of Multicultural Counseling and Development, 32,* 44–61.

Nadal, K. L. (2011). *Filipino American psychology: A handbook of theory, research, and clinical practice.* New York: Wiley.

Nadal, K. L., Rivera, D. P., & Corpus, M. J. H. (2010). Sexual orientation and transgender microaggressions in everyday life: Experiences of lesbians, gays, bisexuals, and transgender individuals. In D. W. Sue (Ed.), *Microaggressions and marginality: Manifestation, dynamics, and impact* (pp. 217–240). New York: Wiley.

Nadal, K. L., & Sue, D. W. (2009). Asian American youth. In C. S. Clauss-Ehlers (Ed.), *Encyclopedia of cross-cultural school psychology* (pp. 116–122). New York: Springer.

Reeves, T. M., & Bennett, C. E. (2004). We the people: Asians in the United States. U.S. Census Bureau, Census 2000 Special Reports. Retrieved on January 31, 2011, from http://www.census.gov/prod/2004pubs/censr-17.pdf.

Root, M. P. P. (1997). Contemporary mixed-heritage Filipino Americans: Fighting colonized identities. In M. P. P. Root (Ed.), *Filipino Americans: Transformation and identity* (pp. 80–94). Thousand Oaks, CA: Sage.

Troiden, R. R. (1989). The formation of homosexual identities. *Journal of Homosexuality, 17,* 43–73.

Appendix: Organizations Dealing with Sexual Victimization and Discrimination of Women

Michele A. Paludi

The following is a listing of resources dealing with sexual victimization of women. This listing serves as a starting point for individuals, family members, and therapists seeking additional information about the sexual victimization of women, including intimate partner violence, rape, sexual harassment, child sexual abuse, stalking, and bullying. This listing is neither complete nor exhaustive. These resources are not to be viewed as substitutes for counseling or for legal advice.

ORGANIZATIONS

Adults and Children Together Against Violence: http://actagainstviolence.apa.org/

Advocates for Youth: http://www.advocatesforyouth.org/about/ywoclc.htm

American Association of University Women: www.aauw.org

American Bar Association Commission on Domestic Violence: www.abanet.org/domviol/home.html

American Domestic Violence Crisis Line: www.awoscentral.com

American Psychological Association: www.apa.org

Antistalking Website: www.antistalking.com

Anti-Violence Resource Guide: http://www.feminist.com/antiviolence/online.html

Asian Task Force Against Domestic Violence: www.atask.org

Asian and Pacific Islander Institute on Domestic Violence: www.apiahf.org/apidvinstitute

Battered Women's Justice Project: www.bwjp.org

Break the Cycle: http://www.breakthecycle.org

British Columbia Institute Against Family Violence: www.bcifv.org

California Coalition Against Sexual Assault: http://calcasa.org

Center for the Study and Prevention of Violence: http://www.colorado.edu/cspv/

Centers for Disease Control and Prevention: www.cdc.gov

Child Find of America: http://www.childfindofamerica.org

Choose Respect: www.chooserespect.org

Coalition Against Trafficking of Women: www.catwinternational.org

Domestic Violence Clearinghouse and Legal Hotline: www.stoptheviolence.org

Equal Employment Opportunity Commission: www.eeoc.gov

Equal Rights Advocates: www.equalrights.org

Family Violence Prevention Fund: www.endabuse.org

Feminist Majority Foundation: www.feminist.org

Girls Inc.: http://www.girlsinc.org/index.html

Institute on Domestic Violence in the African American Community: www.dvinstitute.org

Liz Claiborne: Love Is Not Abuse: http://www.loveisnotabuse.com

MADE (Moms and Dads for Education to Stop Teen Dating Abuse): www.loveisnotabuse.com/made/

Men Can Stop Rape: www.mencanstoprape.org

Mothers Against Teen Violence: http://www.matvinc.org

Ms. Foundation for Women: www.ms.foundation.org

National Center for Victims of Crime: www.ncvc.org

National Center on Elder Abuse: www.ncea.aoa.gov

National Center for Missing and Exploited Children: www.missingkids.com

National Center for Victims of Crime: http://www.ncyc.org

National Coalition Against Domestic Violence: www.ncadv.org

National Domestic Violence Hotline: http://www.ndvh.org

National Institute for Occupational Safety and Health: www.niosh.gov

National Latino Alliance for the Elimination of Domestic Violence: www.dvalianza.org

National Organization for Men Against Sexism: www.nomas.org

National Organization for Women: www.now.org

National Runaway Hotline: http://www.nrscrisisline.org

National Sexual Violence Resource Center: www.nsvrc.org

National Teen Dating Abuse Helpline: http://www.loveisrespect.org

National Women's Law Center: www.nwic.org

National Youth Violence Prevention Resources Center: www.safeyouth.org

Occupational Safety and Health Association: www.osha.gov

Office of Violence Against Women, United States Department of Justice: www.ojp.usdoj.gov

Polly Klaas Foundation: http://www.pollyklaas.org

Prevent Cyberbullying and Internet Harassment: www.cyberbully411.com

Preventing Violence in our Schools: www.extension.umn.edu

Promote Truth: www.promotetruth.org

Rape, Abuse and Incest National Network: www.rainn.org

Safe at Work Coalition: www.safeatworkcoalition.org

Security on Campus: www.securityoncampus.org

Stalking Resource Center: www.ncvc.org/src/Main.aspx

Striving to Reduce Youth Violence Everywhere: http://www.safeyouth.gov/Pages/Home.aspx

Students Against Violence Everywhere: www.nationalsave.org

Teen Dating Violence: http://www.coolnurse.com/teen_dating_violence.html

United Nations Commission on the Status of Women: www.un.org/womenwatch/daw/csw

United Nations Division for the Advancement of Women: www.un.org/womenwatch

United States Department of Education, Office for Civil Rights: www.ed.gov

Womenslaw: http://www.womenslaw.org

Index

Abuse
    physical abuse, 135
    psychological abuse, 135
    sexual abuse, 135
    See also Abuse in adulthood; Child sexual abuse (CSA)
Abuse in adulthood
    batterer intervention programs (BIPs), 127–129
        anger management, 128
        couples counseling, 128
        the Duluth Model, 127
        psychodynamic treatment, 128
    intervention for abusive teens, 129–131
    the likelihood that abusive men will continue to be violent, 125–127
    mental health consequences and correlates of, 121–123
    prevention of, 124
    treatment of abuse survivors, 123–124
    young aggressors becoming adult abusers, 124–125
    See also Adult sexual abuse (ASA)
Adams, J. A., 146
Adult sexual abuse (ASA), 36
    and HIV/AIDS, 45
Aging, double standard for, xxii
Agronick, G., 125

Ahrens, C. E., 9
AIDS. *See* HIV/AIDS
Alcohol-use disorder (AUD), 33
Aldarondo, E., 126
Allstate Insurance Company, SAFE HANDS network, 82
American Bar Association Commission on Domestic Violence, 76
Anatoni, M. H., 46
Angelini, P. J., 25
Arata, C., 36
Armistead, L., 46
Atkins, M. S., 29
Avery-Leaf, S., 129
Axsom, D., 5

Babcock, J., 123, 127, 128
Bakken, T., 108
Bandura, Albert, 141
Banyard, V., 129, 143, 149–150, 150
Barickman, R., 81
Barnes, A., 115
Bauman, K., 125
Bay-Cheng, L. Y., 65
Beezley, D. A., 6
Belle, D., xix
Benefield, T., 125
Bennice, J., 123
Beres, M. A., 55

Berk, R., 104
Bernstein, M., 113, 114
Betz, N. E., 9
Bigler, R., 93
Billingham, R. E., 137
Birns, B., 78
Blaustein, M., 31
Boekeloo, B., 145
Bohmer, S., 142
Borderline personality disorder (BPD), 33–34
Bottoms, B. L., 108
Bowlby, J., 142
Brofenbrenner, U., 143
Bravo-Rosewater, L., xxiv–xxv
Broverman, D., xvii–xviii
Broverman, I., xvii–xviii
Brown, C., 93, 95
Brown, F. A., 58
Brown, J., 146
Brown, Laura S., xvii, xix
Browne, A., 24, 26–27, 30, 32, 34, 36, 37, 44–45
Brownridge, D., 58
Brussat, F., xvi
Brussat, M., xvi
Bryant, C., 73
Buka, S. L., 29, 31–32, 32
Bunch, Charlotte, 17
Burgess, A., 2
Burt, M., 7–8
Butts Stahly, G., 78
Byers, E. S., 24, 36, 37, 58

Callahan, E. D., 34
Canady, B., 123
Capodilupo, C. M., 90
Carey, P. D., 24
Carino, A., 59
Carvalhal, A., 47
Caspi, A., 125
Cavalier, Barbara, 72, 73
Cavalier, Chris, 72
Centers for Disease Control and Prevention, 3, 74, 135
Chapleau, K. M., 8
Chen, H., 146
Cheng, Z., 110

Chesler, Phyllis, xv, xvii
Chien, N. C., 146
Child Abuse and Prevention and Treatment Act (CAPTA), 24
Child Maltreatment 2010 (U.S. Department of Health and Human Services), 25–26
Child sexual abuse (CSA), 24, 38
  defining the problem, 24–25
  and HIV/AIDS, 44–46
  lasting effects of, 29–38
    affective disorders, 32
    anxiety disorders, 29–32
    personality factors, 33–35
    revictimization, 36–37
    sexual identity concerns, 37–38
    somaticism, 35–36
    substance abuse, 32–33
  prevalence of, 25–26
  and PTSD, 29–32
  traumagenic model of, 26–29, 34
    betrayal, 27
    powerlessness (or disempowerment), 27–28
    stigmatization, 28
    traumatic sexualization, 27, 34, 37
Children in Communities Study, 130
Chung, Y. B., 115
Cixous, H., xvii
Clarkson, F., xvii–xviii
Clay, K. M., 32
Clay, S. W., 32
Cleveland, H. H., 146
Cogan, J. C., 110
Cohen, L. L., 91
Cohen, P., 146
Colonial mentality, 169–170
Combs-Lane, A. M., 36
Coping strategies, 13–14, 31
  cognitive coping strategies, 31
  disengagement, 31
  negative coping strategies, 48
  problem-focused coping strategies, 48
Corliss, H. L., 116
Cornwall, J. M., 112
Corporate Alliance to End Partner Violence, 71, 74, 79, 83
Cortina, L. M., 25, 30

Council of Representatives of the American Psychological Association, xxiv
Craig, K. M., 107, 108
Craig, M. E., 57
Cross, C., 129, 143, 149–150, 150
Crow, S. M., 114
Cyr, M., 147

Davidson, J. R. T., 33
Deblinger, E., 29
DeFour, D. C., xxi, xxiii
Des Jardins, K., 74
Diagnostic and Statistical Manual of Mental Disorders, 4th ed. (*DSM-IV-TR*), 28, 29
DiClemente, R. J., 150
DiNitto, D. M., 114
Discrimination, 88
  and identity, 170–171
Dodd, V. J. N., 142
Downing, N. E., 95–96, 166–167
Dubner, A. E., 29
Dunbar, E., 109, 113, 115
Dunner, D. L., 32
Duran, R., 125
Dutton, D. G., 143

East, P. L., 146
Eating disorders, 92
Edmond, T., 15
Ehrensaft, M., 125, 130, 130–131, 146
Eliseo-Arras, R. K., 65
Ellen, J., 49
Ennet, S., 125
Ephross, P., 115
Erotophilia, 37
Erotophobia, 37
Espelage, D. L., 150
Evans, L., 4

FBI
  categories of hate crimes, 105
  statistics on hate crimes, 105–106
  statistics on sexual orientation hate crimes, 109, 110
  Uniform Crime Reporting (UCR) Program, 106

Feerick, M. M., 30
Feinauer, L., 28, 34
Feld, S., 125–126
Feminist identity development model (Downing and Roush), 95–96, 166–167
Feminist therapies, xxiii–xxiv
  and the counseling of rape victims, 15
  guidelines for, xxiv
Feminization of poverty, xix
Ferfusson, D., 125
Filipina American Feminist Identity Development Model, 163–165, 167–170, 168 (table)
Filipino American Identity Development Model, 165–166
Filson, J., 149
Fine, M., 11
Finkelhor, D., 24, 26–27, 30, 32, 34, 36, 37, 44–45
Finkelman, L., 58
Fiske, S. T., 91
Foa, E. B., 29
Fok, L. Y., 114
Forehand, R., 46
Forquer, E. E., 97
Foshee, V., 125, 137, 152
Fourth United Nations International Conference on Women, 74
Foy, D., 30
"Fragment of an Analysis of a Case of Hysteria" (Freud), Dora/Ida in, xvi–xvii
Franklin, K., 107, 112
Freedman, S. D., 32
Freedner, N., 111
Freud, Sigmund, xvi–xvii
Fukuda-Parr, S., xix

Gavey, N., 63, 64–65
Gelles, R., 73
Gender formation, 92–94
Gender norms, 61–62
Gender roles, 90
  and gender role expectations, 94
Gibson, L. E., 31, 36
Gillis, R. J., 110
Glick, P., 91

Glunt, E. K., 110
Goetz, A. T., 60
Gondolf, E., 127
Goodman, L. A., 4
Gottman, J., 126–127
Gover, A. R., 145
Graham, D., 77
Gray, H. M., 137
Green, C., 127
Gregory, D., xix
Grothues, C., 78
Grusky, O., 49
Guidelines for Psychotherapy with Lesbian, Gay, and Bisexual Clients, xxiv
Gwartney-Gibbs, P. A., 142

Haegerich, T., 108
Hall, D. E., 66
Hamilton, J., xix
Harned, M. S., 58
Harrington, K., 150
Harris, D. A., 63
Hartman, S. J., 114
Harvey, M. R., 10
Hate crimes, 103–104
　alternative terms for, 104
　definition of, 104–105
　effects of, 114–115
　FBI categories of, 105
　hate crime legislation
　　Church Arson Prevention Act (1996), 107
　　Civil Rights Law (1964), 106
　　Hate Crime Statistics Act (1990), 106
　　Hate Crimes Sentencing Enhancement Act (1994), 107
　　Matthew Shepard and James Byrd, Jr. Hate Crime Prevention Act (2009), 104, 107
　　reactions to, 107–108
　LGBT hate crimes, 109–110
　　by colleagues/at work, 112–113
　　effects of, 115–116
　　in the family/home, 110–111
　　by peers/in school, 111–112
　　by society, 113
　prevalence of in the United States, 105–106
　reasons for the occurrence of, 104
　sexual orientation hate crimes, 108–109
　effects of, 114–115
Hebert, M., 144, 145, 147–148
Heilbrun, C., xxii
Heise, L., 4
Herd, P., xix
Herek, G. M., 109, 110, 111, 113, 114
Herrenkohl, T., 124
Heterosex, 61
Heymann, J., xx–xxi
Hickman, L. J., 138
Hilton, A., 59
Hilton, G. H., 28, 32, 34
Himelein, M. J., 58
Hines, D. A., 59
HIV/AIDS
　case study, 43–44
　counseling women with HIV/AIDS, 47–50
　and CSA, 44–46
　and experiences with discrimination, 46–47
Hokoda, A., 144, 146, 149, 152
Holland, J., 62
Holloway, W., 61
Holmstrom, L., 2
Holt, M. K., 150
Horne, S., 74
Horvath, M., 112
Horwood, L., 125
Howard, D. E., 145
Huang, B., 124
Humphrey, J. A., 25
Hyde, A., 62, 65
Hysteria, xvii
Hyun, M., 32

Identity, and discrimination, 170–171
Ingram, K., 9
Intimate partner violence, 73
　behaviors that suggest intimate partner violence, 76
　emotional/psychological effects of, 77
　female victims of, 73–74
　impact of on organizations, 74–75
　impact of on social and interpersonal relationships, 77

impact of on victims, 75–78
implications for parenting, 77
physical/health-related effects of, 76–77
why women remain in violent relationships, 77–78
and the workplace, 71–74, 78–83
  consensual relationship policy, 80–81
  effective prevention programs, 82
  employee assistance program (EAP) counselors, 81
  engineering solutions (safety plans), 79–80
  policies and procedures, 79
  training programs, 79
  See also Intimate partner violence during adolescence
Intimate partner violence during adolescence
  consequences of, 148–150
    educational outcomes, 149–150
    mental health concerns, 148–149
    revictimization, 149
  definitions of, 135–137
  intervention and prevention programs, 150–152
  intimate partner violence theories
    attachment theory, 142–143
    feminist theory, 141
    social learning theory, 141–142
    socioecological model, 143–144
  perpetrators/victims of, 137–138
  prevalence of, 138–140
  risk factors
    contextual factors, 147–148
    environmental factors, 146–147
    individual factors, 145–146
    sociodemographic factors, 144–145
  and social support, 150

Jackson, S., 128
Jacobson, N., 126–127
Janoff-Bulman, R., 11
Johnson, J. G., 146
Jones, L. M., 26
Jordan, C., 4

Kaestle, C. E., 59
Kahn, A. S., 5
Kaiser Permanente, 82
Kaniasty, K., 16
Katz, J., 57, 58, 59
Keeping Children and Families Safe Act (2003), 24
Kempley, R., xv
Kendall-Tackett, K. A., 30, 38
Kendler, K. S., 29, 33
Kessler, R. C., 29, 31–32, 32
Kilpatrick, D. G., 36
Kimerling, R., 46
King, Rodney, 107
Knefel, A., 73
Knight, R. A., 63
Knight, W. G., 31
Koss, M. P., 4, 6, 10
Kostelac, C., 113, 114
Koverola, C., 30
Krahe, B., 6, 7
Kristensen, E., 35
Kubiak, S. P., 25, 30
Kuffel, S. W., 58

Lamb, S., 15
Landecker, H., 34
Lang, D. L., 150
Lau, M., 35
Lavin-Loucks, D., xix
Lavoie, F., 58
Lawrence, F. M., 104–106
Leaper, C., 95
Lees, S., 6
Leitenberg, H., 31
Lemeiux, S. R., 24, 36, 37
Leonard, K. E., 6, 126
Leonard, L., 49
Lerman, Hannah, xxiii
Lerner, M. J., 8
Lewin, M., 5
Littleton, H., 5
Liu, H., 45
Liz Claiborne, 74, 79, 82
Lloyd, S., 77
Locus of control (LOC), external, 33
Logan, T. K., 4, 75, 76
Long, P. J., 45

Longfellow, C., xix
Lonsway, K., 16
Lott, B., 6

Macke, C., 76
Magdol, L., 125, 130, 145, 146
Magruder, B., 60
Maier, A., 146
Makosky, V., xix
Mannison, M., 57
Marecek, J., xxi
Marmion, S., 78
Martin, C., 93
Martin, M., xix
Martin del Campo, M. A., 144
Matheson, K., 58
Mathie, V. A., 5
McDevitt, J., 114–115
McGregor, J., 55
McHugh, M. C., 6
McLeer, S. V., 29
McMullin, D., 25
McNally, R. J., 30
McNaughton Reyes, H., 152
McPhail, B. A., 104, 114
Mental health, double standard for, xvii–xviii
Messman-Moore, T. L., 45
Microaggressions, 89
  gender microaggressions, 90, 91–92
    assumptions of inferiority, 90
    assumptions of traditional gender roles, 90
    denial of individual sexism, 90
    denial of reality of sexism, 90
    environmental microaggressions, 90
    second-class citizenship, 90
    sexist language, 90
    sexual objectification, 90, 94–95
  influences of intersectional identities, 96–97, 98
  racial microaggressions, 97
    alien in one's own land, 97
    assumption of criminality, 97
  responses of victims to, 89
  sexual orientation/transgender microaggressions, 97–98
    assumption of sexual pathology or abnormality, 97–98
    discomfort/disapproval of LGBT experience, 97
Middleton, K. C., 28
Mikel Brown, L., 140
Milburn, M. A., 63
Miller, A. J., 112
Miller, C., 93
Mindes, E. J., 9
Modecki, K. L., 143
Model minority myth, 164
Moffitt, T., 125
Mohr, N., 24
Molnar, B. E., 31–32, 32
Motley, M. T., 63
Motta, R. W., 29
Muehlenhard, C., 6
Mulder, R., 29
Myers, H., 45, 48
Myhr, I., 57
Myint-U, A., 125

Nadal, K. L., 90, 164
Nation, T., 152
National Coalition of Anti-Violence Programs, 108
National College Health Risk Behavior Survey, 1
National Comorbidity Survey (NCS), 29, 31
National Crime Victimization Survey (NCVS), 3, 139
National Family Violence Survey, 125–126
National Institute for Occupational Health and Safety, 73
National Violence Against Women Survey, 1, 3, 122
Nelson, S., 35–36
Ng, M. T., 45, 48
Nightmares
  Type I, 30
  Type II, 30
Norris, F., 16
Nuts (Topor), Claudia Draper in, xv–xvi, xvii
Nydegger, R., 79, 80

Obama, Barack, 104
Occupational Safety Act, 78
Occupational Safety and Health
   Administration, 73, 78, 82
O'Donnell, L., 125
Offman, A., 58
O'Keefe, M., 141–142, 142
O'Leary, D., 126
O'Leary, K. D., 59, 138
Olsheski, J. A., 32
Oros, C. J., 6
O'Sullivan, L. F., 58, 64
Oswald, D. L., 8

Paludi, C., 79, 80
Paludi, M., xxi, xxii–xxiii, 79, 80, 81
Partnership for Prevention, 81
Patton, W., 57
Paymar, M., 127
Peel, F., 113
Pence, E., 127
Peters, S. D., 25
Poitras, M., 58
Polakoff, E., xix
Post-traumatic growth (PTG), 12–13
   components of, 12
   estimated prevalence rates for, 12
   other terms used for, 12
Post-traumatic stress disorder (PTSD), 10, 27, 28, 122
   and CSA, 29–32
Poteat, V. P., 116
Putnam, F., 46
Putnam, S. E., 30

Qui, Y., 145
Quigley, B., 126

Ragins, B. R., 113
Ralph, D. L., 29
Rangel, R., 97
Rape
   comparison with verbal sexual coercion, 54–56
   definition of, 3
   and ethnicity, 4
   impact of on women's lives, 2
   mental health effects, 10–12
   physical health impacts, 9–10
   interventions with rape victims, 14–15
   personal growth and coping following rape, 12–14
   prevalence and persistence of, 1–2
   prevention of, 16–17
   and rape myths, 7–8, 16
   rape crisis centers, 15
   and the rape trauma syndrome, 2
   and the sexual double standard, 6
   and sexual scripts, 5–6
   sociocultural conceptions of, 2–3
   and victim blame, 8–9
   and vulnerability, 4
Rawlings, E., 77
Reinholtz, C., 25
Renner, L., 137
Resnick, H. S., 36
Revised Conflict Tactics Scales (CTS2), 58–59
Reyes, L., 25
Rich, C. L., 36, 149
Ridley, E., 76
Rivera, D. P., 97
Roberts, A., 127
Roberts, K. J., 49
Roberts, T. A., 146
Robie, C., 127
Roosa, M. W., 25
Roper, A., 81
Rosenkrantz, P., xvii–xviii
Roush, K. L., 95–96, 166–167
Rozee, P. D., 2, 3, 5, 5–6, 16, 17
Ruble, D. N., 83
Runfola, C., 149
Russo, N. F., xviii, 4
Ryan, A. M., 112

Safe Horizon, 74, 79
Salazar, L. F., 150
Saltzburg, S., 110
Sanday, P., 3
Saunders, E., xix
Saudino, K. J., 59
Savage, S. A., 146
Schatzel-Murphy, E., 63
Schmitt, M. M., 9
Schulhofer, S. J., 55

Schwartz, M., 129
Seal, D. W., 63, 65–66
Secondary victimization. *See* Victim blaming
Seedat, S., 24
Sexism, 88–89
  forms of
    benevolent sexism, 91
    covert sexism, 91
    hostile sexism, 91
    overt sexism, 91
    subtle sexism, 91
  influence of on mental health and development, 92–96
  sexist language, 90
  See also Microaggressions
Sexual assault. *See* Rape
Sexual autonomy, 55
Sexual behavior, double standard for, 6–7
Sexual Coercion in Intimate Relationships Scale (SCIR), 60
Sexual consent, 55, 65–66
Sexual Experiences Survey (SES), 57–58
Sexual objectification, 90, 94–95
Sexual scripts, 5–6, 62, 62–64, 64
Shackelford, T. K., 60
Showalter, E., xvi–xvii
Silva, P., 125
Simoni, J. M., 45, 48
Sims, E. N., 142
Smailes, E., 146
Smith, N. G., 9
Smith, P. H., 149
Smith Slep, A. M., 138
Snow, K. L., 30
Speech, L., 79
Spinazzola, J., 31
Stein, D. J., 24
Steinmetz, S., 73
Stevenson, E., 4
Stockard, J., 142
Straus, M., 73, 125–126
Straus, M. A., 146
Struckman-Johnson, C., 59–60
Stueve, A., 125
Suchindran, C., 125

Sue, D. W., 172
Sullivan, H., 6
Summer, Lawrence, 94
Sun, K., 104
Swanberg, J., 75, 76, 79
Swanson, A. N., 49
Swim, J. K., 91
Szymanski, D. M., 116

Taft, C., 123
Tajima, E., 124
Taluc, N., 77
Tartaro, J., xviii
Tejeda, M. J., 142
Terr, L. C., 30
Teten, A. L., 138
Thibos, M., xix
Thoennes, N., 74
Tjaden, P., 74
Topor, Tom, xv
Torgler, C., 5
Tran, C., 74
Traumatic sexualization, 27, 34, 37
Tyra, P. A., 15

Ueno, K., 115
Ulloa, E. C., 144, 147, 149
Ulman, S. E., 8–9, 15
U.S. Census Bureau, 88
U.S. Department of Health and Human Services, 25
U.S. Department of Justice
  Bureau of Justice Statistics, 139
  Office of Violence Against Women, 3
U.S. Department of Labor, Bureau of Labor Statistics, xx
U.S. Equal Employment Opportunity Commission, 99

van der Kolk, B. A., 31, 33
Vanderhaar, Gerard, 78
VanderLaan, D. P., 62
Vasey, P. L., 62
Verbal sexual coercion, 53–54, 66–67
  comparison with rape, 54–56
  and the CTS2, 58–59
  and gender norms in heterosexual context, 61–62

prevalence of in young adult
heterosexual relationships, 57
research on not using CTS2 or SES,
59–60
responses to verbal coercion, 64–65
and the SES, 57–58
and sexual consent in relational context,
65–66
sexual initiation and coercion, 62–64
terms used for, 54
verbal tactics used, 54–55
Vezina, J., 144, 145, 147–148
Victim blaming, 8–9, 56
implicit blaming, 8
overt blaming, 8
Violent Crime Control and Law
Enforcement Act (1994), 106
Vogel, R. E., 58
Vogel, S., xvii–xviii

Waldner-Haugrud, L. K., 60
Waldo, C. R., 108, 112–113
Walker, J. L., 24, 32
Walker, L., 77, 122
Walsh, K., 31
Warshaw, C., 122, 123–124
Watson, B., 6
Wetterstein, K., 75
White, J. W., 25
White, S., xix
Whitney, S., 124, 137
Williams, J., xvii

Williams, M. C., 59
Williams, T., 115
Willis, D. G., 109
Willman, S., 75
Wilmot, J., 79
Wilson-Simmons, R., 125
Wingood, G. M., 46, 150
Wirth, R. J., 25
Women, and mental disorders
diagnosis and treatment of, xviii–xix
impact of violence on, xxii–xxiii
older women and mental health issues,
xxi–xxii
and stressors involved in multiple roles
of women, xx–xxi
and stressors involved in poverty, xix
Woodward, L., 125
Worell, J., xxiv
Workplace violence, 73
female victims of, 73
male victims of, 73
See also Intimate partner violence, and
the workplace
World Health Organization, 3
Wyatt, G. E., 4, 25, 45

Yang, A. S., 110, 112, 113
Yonkers, K., xix
Youth Risk Behavior Surveillance System
(YRBSS), 139

Zelkowitz, P., xix

About the Editors and Contributors

EDITORS

PAULA K. LUNDBERG-LOVE is a professor of psychology at the University of Texas at Tyler (UTT) and was the Ben R. Fisch Endowed Professor in Humanitarian Affairs for 2001–2004. Her undergraduate degree was in chemistry, and she worked as a chemist at a pharmaceutical company for five years prior to earning her doctorate in physiological psychology with an emphasis in psychopharmacology. After a three-year postdoctoral fellowship in nutrition and behavior in the Department of Preventive Medicine at the Washington University School of Medicine in St. Louis, she assumed her academic position at UTT, where she teaches classes in psychopharmacology, behavioral neuroscience, physiological psychology, sexual victimization, and family violence. Subsequent to her academic appointment, Dr. Lundberg-Love pursued postgraduate training and is a licensed professional counselor. She is a member of the Tyler Counseling and Assessment Center, where she provides therapeutic services for victims of sexual assault, child sexual abuse, and domestic violence. She has conducted a long-term research study on women who were victims of childhood incestuous abuse, constructed a therapeutic program for their recovery, and documented its effectiveness on their recovery. She is the author of nearly 100 publications and presentations and is coeditor of *Violence and Sexual Abuse at Home: Current Issues in Spousal Battering and Child Maltreatment* as well as *Intimate Violence against Women: When Spouses, Partners, or Lovers Attack*. As a result of her training in psychopharmacology and child maltreatment, her expertise has been sought as a consultant on various death penalty appellate cases in the state of Texas.

KEVIN L. NADAL, PhD, is an assistant professor of psychology and mental health counseling at the John Jay College of Criminal Justice–City University of

New York and earned his doctorate in counseling psychology from Columbia University. He has published several works focusing on Filipino American, ethnic minority, and LGBT issues in the fields of psychology and education. He is a fellow of the Robert Wood Johnson Foundation and is the author of the books *Filipino American Psychology: A Handbook of Theory, Research, and Clinical Practice* and *Filipino American Psychology: A Collection of Personal Narratives*.

MICHELE A. PALUDI, PhD, is the series editor for Women's Psychology and for Women and Careers in Management for Praeger. She is the author/editor of 38 college textbooks and of more than 170 scholarly articles and conference presentations on sexual harassment, campus violence, psychology of women, gender, and discrimination. Her book *Ivory Power: Sexual Harassment on Campus* (1990, SUNY Press) received the 1992 Myers Center Award for Outstanding Book on Human Rights in the United States. Dr. Paludi served as chair of the U.S. Department of Education's Subpanel on the Prevention of Violence, Sexual Harassment, and Alcohol and Other Drug Problems in Higher Education. She was one of six scholars in the United States to be selected for this subpanel. She also was a consultant to and a member of former New York State governor Mario Cuomo's Task Force on Sexual Harassment. Dr. Paludi serves as an expert witness for court proceedings and administrative hearings on sexual harassment. She has had extensive experience in conducting training programs and investigations of sexual harassment and other Equal Employment Opportunity (EEO) issues for businesses and educational institutions. In addition, Dr. Paludi has held faculty positions at Franklin & Marshall College, Kent State University, Hunter College, Union College, and Union Graduate College, where she directs the human resource management certificate program. She is on the faculty in the School of Management. She was selected as the Elihu Root Visiting Professor of Women's Studies at Hamilton College for fall, 2011. She was recently named "Woman of the Year" by the Business and Professional Women in Schenectady, New York.

CONTRIBUTORS

DONNA CASTAÑEDA, PhD, is a professor in the Psychology Department at San Diego State University–Imperial Valley. She completed her BA in psychology at the University of Washington and her MA and PhD in social psychology at the University of California, Davis. Dr. Castañeda has investigated the impact of close relationship factors in HIV sexual risk behavior, particularly among Latinos; the HIV/AIDS prevention needs of women factory workers in Mexico; and the close relationship context and how it affects intimate partner violence and the relationship between mental health and marital satisfaction. A second area of interest is the role of structural factors or aspects of service delivery systems in the provision of health and mental health services to Latina/Latino communities.

DESIREE L. GLAZE is a graduate student in the MS Clinical Psychology program at the University of Texas at Tyler (UT-Tyler), where she anticipates graduating in December 2011. While at UT-Tyler she has participated in research projects. Her academic goals include becoming a licensed professional counselor and obtaining a doctorate in psychology. She wants to conduct research with and provide therapeutic intervention for children who have experienced sexual abuse. She is a 2009 graduate of Abilene Christian University in Abilene, Texas, where she earned a BS in psychology. While an undergraduate, she was accepted as a member of Psi Chi, the national honor society in psychology; served as a research assistant; and was a member of Abilene Christian University Honor's Program.

KATIE E. GRIFFIN is a recent graduate of CUNY John Jay College's master's in forensic psychology program. She has worked on various research projects involving racial, sexual orientation, and religious microaggressions under the advisement of Kevin L. Nadal, PhD, and her thesis project focused on individuals' empathy levels for victims of hate crimes. Currently she is a statistics lab coordinator and an adjunct professor at CUNY John Jay College teaching undergraduate criminal justice and statistic courses. She continues to do qualitative and quantitative research on microaggressions as a member of Dr. Nadal's research team. Katie plans to pursue her PhD in forensic or social psychology and use her background in microaggressions and hate crimes research to assist her in doctoral-level study.

KRISTAL HAYNES has her bachelor of science in psychology from Messiah College and is a PhD student at CUNY Graduate Center studying developmental psychology. Her research focuses on minority youth development and women's issues. She currently works at John Jay College as a research assistant studying the physical and mental health of Filipino American youths, as directed by Dr. Kevin Nadal.

AUDREY HOKODA, PhD, is an associate professor in the Child and Family Development Department at San Diego State University. She received her BS in psychobiology from the University of California, Los Angeles, and her doctorate in clinical psychology from the University of Illinois, Urbana Champaign. She has been the principal investigator for more than 15 studies and community projects focused on developing, implementing, and evaluating youth violence prevention programs. Her primary areas of research are peer abuse, teen relationship violence, and children's exposure to domestic violence.

JENNIFER KATZ, PhD, is a licensed psychologist and an associate professor of psychology at SUNY College at Geneseo in upstate New York. Her research interests focus on the sociocultural context of individual mental health, with a particular emphasis on couple relationships, intimate partner violence, and sexual coercion.

KELLY A. KOVACK is a clinical psychology doctoral student at Indiana University of Pennsylvania. Her research interests include various forms of trauma, post-traumatic growth, coping, and negative social support. Her clinical work has included inpatient and outpatient therapy and assessment with individuals facing issues such as chronic mental illness, post-traumatic stress, traumatic brain injury, and substance abuse. Her doctoral research focuses on post-traumatic growth.

MAUREEN C. McHUGH is a social psychologist and gender specialist. A professor of psychology at Indiana University of Pennsylvania, she has introduced more than 2,500 students to the psychology of women. In addition to journal articles, McHugh has published 20 chapters, many in edited texts focused on the psychology of women including the first *Handbook on the Psychology of Women*. Her work focuses on gender differences, feminist methods, and violence against women. She is currently working on intimate partner violence, street harassment, and slut bashing. McHugh served as the president equivalent of the Association for Women in Psychology (AWP) and received the Christine Ladd Franklin Award for service to the AWP and feminist psychology. For her work with both graduate and undergraduate women, she was honored with the Florence Denmark Distinguished Mentoring Award.

WESLEY S. PARKS is a graduate student at the University of Texas in Tyler, where he is soon to complete a master's degree in clinical psychology with a specialization in neuropsychology. His undergraduate degree also was in psychology. For the past five years he has worked at a private forensic and clinical psychology practice in the Dallas–Fort Worth Metroplex, where he has been involved in wide-ranging and often high-profile forensic psychology and legal cases. His burgeoning research interests include effects of exposure to traumatic events, business and organizational psychology, the role of psychology in shaping public policy, affective disorders, and jury selection and groupthink in capital murder trials.

JULIE RAMOS is a graduate of the master's program in forensic mental counseling at the John Jay College of Criminal Justice, City University of New York. Her clinical experience has been with an array of populations including women with HIV/AIDS, substance abusers, and victims of intimate partner violence.

DAVID A. SCHUBERTH is a current master's student in CUNY John Jay College's forensic psychology program and an alumnus of Clark University. He has worked on a number of research projects that have involved topics such as acculturation, conformity to gender norms, psychopathy, eyewitness accuracy, and secondary victims of homicide. His current thesis project will focus on the role of empathy in moral judgments expressed by college students with varying levels of psychopathic personality characteristics. Other ongoing research projects include an examination of psychopathic traits and possible protective factors found in police and other hero populations. David plans to pursue a PhD in clinical psychology and will be using his diverse background in various types of research to assist in doctoral-level study.

MELANIE SCHUKRAFFT is an undergraduate student at SUNY Geneseo. Her research interests focus on young adult sexual development, including understanding responses to partner violence and sexual coercion.

About the Editors and Contributors

WILLIAM E. SCHWEINLE received his doctorate in 2002 from the University of Texas at Arlington, majoring in social and quantitative psychology. He received postdoctoral training in quantitative psychology at the University of Missouri–Columbia. Dr. Schweinle has studied men's maltreatment of women for 14 years and has published several articles and book chapters on the subject of abusive men's social cognition. He is currently an assistant professor of biostatistics in the University of South Dakota School of Health Sciences.

VANESSA TIRONE is a doctoral student in clinical psychology at the University of Tennessee, Knoxville. Her research interests focus on the impact of sexual victimization and unwanted consensual sex on women's psychological well-being and relationship functioning.

MONICA ULIBARRI is an assistant professor in the Department of Psychiatry at the University of California, San Diego, and a clinical supervisor in the SDSU/UCSD joint doctoral program in clinical psychology. She received her BA in psychology from Claremont McKenna College and her MA and PhD in clinical psychology from Arizona State University. Dr. Ulibarri's research focuses on HIV prevention in the Latino community, with an emphasis on how gender-based violence, mental health, and substance use intersect with HIV risk behaviors.

EMILIO ULLOA, PhD, is the director of undergraduate advising and programs in the Psychology Department at San Diego State University. He completed his BA in psychology at San Diego State University and his MA and PhD in social psychology at Arizona State University. Dr. Ulloa has published research investigating dating or relationship violence among teens and college students, the association between violence and HIV/AIDS risk, and the association between childhood sexual abuse and relationship violence.

BETH A. WATSON is a clinical psychology doctoral student at Indiana University of Pennsylvania. Her research focuses on feminist methods, the sexual double standard, slut bashing, and contraceptive use. Her doctoral research is on the sexual double standard, and she has presented on this regionally and at the Association for Women in Psychology. Her clinical work focuses on outpatient therapy with sexual abuse victims and inpatient therapy and risk evaluations with sexual offenders. Ms. Watson currently teaches as an adjunct faculty member at Westmoreland County Community College.

VANESSA WATTS is a second-year master's student at San Diego State University and in the Teen Relationship Violence Lab. She received her BS from the University of Utah. Her thesis will be on examining the relationship between harmful family dynamics and continuous or repeated dating violence in middle and high school students.